Practical make-up

LINDA MEREDITH

Hodder & Stoughton

A MEMBER OF THE HODDER HEADLINE GROUP

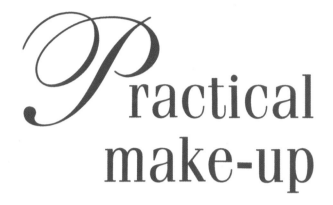

Practical
make-up

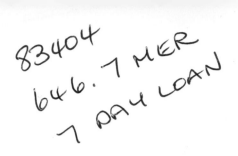
Cataloguing in Publication Data is available from the British Library

ISBN 0 340 59513 2

First published 1994
Impression number   10 9 8 7 6 5 4 3 2 1
Year   1998 1997 1996 1995 1994

Typeset by Wearset, Boldon, Tyne and Wear.
Printed in Hong Kong for Hodder & Stoughton Educational, a division of Hodder Headline Plc, 338 Euston Road, London NW1 3BH by Colorcraft Ltd.

Contents

To my father for instilling in me the importance of education

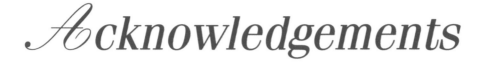

Acknowledgements

I would like to thank Brian Messam, Emily Marcou, Sally Cavanagh and Lily Panic for their invaluable assistance with the hair and make-up featured in this book, Jim Macavoy of Surefil for technical advice, and Christina Jansen for her time, patience and expert photography. I am grateful to Screenface for supplying the cosmetics used and to High Peak for providing the brushes.

In addition, many thanks go to Julie Houlsby, Hiromi Kikukawa, Lily Panic, Syreeta Brown, Kim Kayne, Reena Patel, Dionne Powell, Karin Sang, Kathleen Mason and Nicola Jones for modelling for the photographs.

Lastly, thank you to Pirelli for allowing us to reproduce photographs from the 1992 Pirelli calendar, and to Thomas Blake for supplying the photographs of cosmetic camouflage.

The cosmetics used on the front cover were supplied courtesy of Surefil and Screenface.

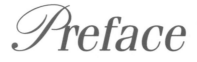

Preface

In writing this book, I have focused on the easiest, most up-to-date techniques and styles of make-up, both for the client and for the professional.

All the methods I use are common practice in industry and will therefore equip students for their professional careers. As a specific guide, at the beginning of each chapter you will find more detail about the NVQ standards for make-up application, as set out below:

Level 1 – Assist the therapist with treatments
Element 1: Prepare the client and cleanse the skin for cosmetic application

Level 2 – Apply and instruct on make-up
Element 1: Cleanse and prepare the client for make-up application
Element 2: Apply make-up to the face
Element 3: Provide advice on self-use of facial make-up and homecare

Level 2 – Provide lash and brow treatments
Element 3: Apply false eyelashes

There are many different fields within the make-up industry. Although I do not profess to be an expert in all of them, I am an authority on the styles of make-up featured in this book. I am a make-up teacher first and foremost and my students are successfully working in all the different fields of make-up. My responsibilities as a teacher dictate that I should also be up to date with methods and techniques as well as the technology relating to the make-up industry. I am constantly trying out new techniques and looking for new styles – any truly professional make-up artist will do the same. Otherwise experience will turn out to be, in the words of a famous American surgeon, doing the same thing over and over again badly.

The techniques and guidelines presented in this book have been tried and tested many times during the 15 years that I have been teaching make-up. I will discuss different methods of application, the textures of products and the tools of the trade. Whichever method you decide to follow is up to you; the most important thing is achieving an end result that you, the client and the professional are happy and confident with.

Introduction

There are many areas where professional make-up artists can demonstrate their skills; film, television, theatre and the glamorous world of photographic and fashion. Some make-up artists are used to design the looks required, while others are employed in the actual application. All these styles of make-up are applied to the professional artist, whether actor or model, which is why professional make-up is classed as being different from the make-up applied in a salon situation.

Most beauty salons do, however, offer a make-up service to their clients, and it is an important area for beauty therapists and hairdressers to master. Even without a natural flair for make-up, a good understanding of the products used and, of course, the techniques with which to apply them will enable any therapist or hairdresser to be confident in offering the client a good professional make-up.

Firstly, it should be understood that salon make-up can create an illusion which will emphasize the good points and disguise the bad ones. What it cannot do is to totally change the shape of the face or magically diminish a double chin or crooked nose. All aspects of salon make-up can be seen at close proximity and, therefore, shading and shaping may only accentuate features that you would otherwise want to minimize.

Secondly, when consulting a client, it is not just the face which should be taken into consideration but also the overall style of the hair and the outfit being worn. For example, two clients of the same age wishing to have the same make-up applied would require a totally different look if one was a business executive and the other a housewife.

The professional make-up artist has the advantage of being able to choose the product he or she wants to work with. By contrast, most beauty salons stock a particular range of cosmetics so that they are able to retail the product as well as to use it in make-up application. After all, a salon is a business and if the make-up is well applied it will most certainly lead to the client purchasing at least some of the products which have been used during the application.

Many clients will have a definite idea of the style of make-up they wish to have, while others will leave it totally to the professional. To assist in this, it is advisable to have a selection of looks and ideas from which the client can choose. Although the choice may not be ideally suited to the client's features, any look can be varied or adapted to suit the individual.

REMEMBER

A good make-up can always be achieved if it is broken down into sections and taken one step at a time.

Preparation

KEY AREAS

By the end of this chapter you will know about:

- Cleansing and preparing the client for make-up application
- Skin cleansing products in relation to skin types
- Dealing with contra-indications

Preparation for salon make-up

Skin

Although not required in professional make-up, Cleanse, Tone and Moisturize has always been an accepted part of the make-up application in a salon.

Cleansing

REMEMBER

All old make-up must be removed before you start work.

Eye make-up should always be removed with a non-oily eye make-up remover. Any oily product around the eye area would cause the newly applied eye make-up to crease or smudge easily. Lipstick pigment will generally stain the skin, especially the more vibrant colours. It is therefore important that all of the colour is removed during cleansing, otherwise residue pigment from the old lipstick could influence the colour of the new one being applied.

Toning

Once the whole face has been cleansed of any remaining make-up, toner or astringent should be used to remove all traces of the cleanser. (Toner is used on a dry skin, astringent on an oily skin.) At this point the skin should be checked over the entire face to make sure that it does not feel tacky, as any residue of cleanser would lead to an uneven base. The skin is now ready to be moisturized.

REMEMBER

Check the skin at regular intervals throughout the make-up. Always use the back of your hand as the palm may be sticky.

Moisturizing

During skin treatments, several different types of moisturizer can be used, depending on the type of skin being treated (dry, oily, combination, etc). It is important, however, that under make-up the moisturizer used is compatible with the make-up, not necessarily with the skin.

REMEMBER

A compatible moisturizer is one that totally absorbs into the skin, leaving no residue on the surface. If excess moisturizer is left on the surface of the skin, it could result in the movement and eventual disappearance of the foundation.

Different textures will absorb into the skin at different rates; some will disappear totally within one minute, while others may take up to four or five. It is important to be aware of the absorption rate of the moisturizer being used. Firstly, check the moisturizer on the back of your own hand to see if it is compatible with make-up at all. Secondly, try a patch test on your client's skin as it may react in a different way. A neutral surface, such as the back of the client's hand, will give you a good indication.

In some salons the Cleanse, Tone and Moisturize is carried out in a facial chair for convenience to the operator. If the client is then taken to the make-up area, be sure to check the moisturizer again before applying the foundation. It may be necessary to apply a second layer if the first has been totally absorbed into the skin. If the basic cleanse is carried out in the make-up area, it will not be necessary to check the moisturizer as the foundation will be applied immediately.

Foundation

This is where you can see how important it is to know and understand the textures of the products being used. The compatibility of the moisturizer with the foundation is vital to the overall blending and durability of the foundation. For example, if a heavy moisturizer is used with a foundation which has a high content of oil, the result will be excessive streaking and the colour products will become patchy and difficult to apply. On the other hand, if a light, highly absorbent moisturizer is used with a foundation which has a high content of water, the foundation will not blend at all. Either extreme would make the application very difficult and would also result in an uncomfortable feeling for the client.

It is tempting to apply the base quickly so that more time can be spent in perfecting the colour products. In practice, however, this is completely the wrong thing to do. The base is the canvas and therefore of vital importance. A perfect foundation is the hardest part of a make-up to achieve as its texture and thickness must be varied on each individual if the overall finish is to look natural. A perfect base ensures that all the colour products will blend without the risk of them becoming patchy or streaky. More importantly, it will also give the final make-up staying power – you can then be confident that the make-up will remain as perfect as when first applied, even up to ten hours later.

Different skin types

It is quite probable that you will also have to apply make-up to extreme skin types; excessively dry or excessively oily. These skin types must be treated beforehand, otherwise they will affect the finish of the foundation.

Dry skin
Any obvious dry areas should be removed with a fine exfoliating cream. Failure to do so would result in an uneven finish, with the foundation appearing thicker on the dry patches.

Oily skin
The skin may be excessively oily down the centre panel or over the entire face. Products (sealer/anti-shine) dealing with this problem are readily available. They allow the skin to produce oil, but create a barrier (generally containing some form of silicone) which does not allow the oil through to lift off the make-up. The products come in different forms and textures – some will dry completely, others will remain tacky like an ordinary moisturizer. If the sealer dries completely, it would be advisable to use a foundation with a higher oil content to allow the movement needed for blending. However, if the foundation used contains more water than oil, an alternative would be to apply a fine layer of moisturizer over the top of the sealer.

Sometimes these products come in the form of a cream, rather like a moisturizer. If the foundation contains a high content of oil, the barrier cream should be allowed to absorb into the skin first to prevent streaking. If the foundation contains a higher water content, use the barrier cream to assist in the blending.

Cosmetic textures will be explained in detail in chapter 2.

Contra-indications

In most areas of beauty therapy, contra-indications must be checked fully before any treatment is given, because of the health and safety factor. When dealing with make-up, however, contra-indications should be looked at from a slightly different perspective. Make-up cannot damage the skin – in fact it can provide protection against the harmful effects of the atmosphere – but it must be removed thoroughly within 24 hours, otherwise the molecules will break down and small particles can absorb through the epidermis.

REMEMBER

Hygiene must be a priority in any make-up application.

Clean brushes and applicators must be used on each client and, where any infections are apparent (such as sores or sties), cosmetic products should be applied from a spatula or palate knife, not taken directly from the make-up. Skin complaints should be dealt with (depending on the severity) by using extra product to conceal them or by using cosmetic camouflage techniques (see chapter 6).

Salon client

The client should always be positioned vertically, as any angle to the body will distort the bone structure and prevent the skin from falling into its normal position. This will be more evident in the older client.

Ideally, the client's head should be level with the make-up artist's shoulder. If for some reason this position is not possible, it is important that the top of the client's head is never lower than the make-up artist's shoulders. In the long run this will prevent neck and back problems for the artist.

Section clips or a very loose headband should be used so that the hairline and the front part of the client's ears are visible. The ears are used as a guideline when blusher is applied. Check the headband – if it is too tight the make-up artist will be unable to blend the edges of the foundation away at the hairline.

A make-up cape or tissues should be used around the client's neckline to protect clothing, leaving (if possible) the chest and arms visible. An off-the-shoulder gown may be worn for a wedding or evening make-up, in which case the make-up artist would need to take the skin tone in those areas into consideration when choosing the correct colour of foundation.

Finally, before any application of products, the eyebrows must be checked and shaped. Well-shaped eyebrows are a very important part of the total make-up – they are the framework for the eyes and form part of the character of the face. The eyes may water during plucking so it is advisable to check them before continuing. (Eyebrow shaping is discussed in detail in chapter 4.)

Salon lighting

Many modern salons designate a specific area for make-up application. Unfortunately, many salon owners are misguided when choosing the correct lighting for this area. It may look professional to have the mirror surrounded by bright lights but, in reality, the amount of heat given off by so many light bulbs will affect the make-up application.

Professional make-up first began in the theatre. These large old buildings were often very cold and the wax products used needed both the warmth of the fingers and the heat from the lights to enable the actor to blend them. By contrast, beauty salons are usually warm places as many of the treatments are carried out with the client undressed. If, in addition, heat is given off by lights which surround the mirror, the fine textures of foundation used today will melt. Cold strip lights are used in professional location mirrors. This type of lighting would also be ideally suited to the warm environment of the beauty salon.

Make-up is applied in a series of stages, rather like a painting. The first stages may look awful but the correct groundwork is vital to the end result. These first stages quickly change once the make-up is finished and the warmth of the body begins to come through. It is for this reason that the client is better positioned with her back to the mirror for a make-up. If a make-up lesson is to be given, the client will have to be positioned facing the mirror. However, more time will then be spent in explaining the changes that take place throughout the make-up.

Ti**P** ●

Daylight can be very deceptive and is in fact much stronger than we realize. Many books and articles on lighting state that daylight is the best light to work in. I totally disagree. I have always found that the best situation to work in is one with as little daylight as possible. If the room has windows, go to the furthest point away from them — you will find the make-up much easier to apply as the light is less likely to create shadows.

● ●

The layout of each salon is obviously different, so the final decision on lighting must be left to the individual make-up artist.

Preparation for professional make-up

Television presenter

Most television studios are well equipped with a make-up area or room in which to prepare the interviewer and guests. As the make-up artist is responsible for the total presentation of each individual, the make-up room should be well equipped with everything that would be needed for the hair as well as the make-up. There should also be an iron, ironing board and a sewing kit in cases of emergency. If the make-up artist is resident in the studio, then it is obviously his or her responsibility to ensure that everything required is on hand. There are, however, very few resident make-up artists working in the industry today, and it is more likely that a freelance make-up artist would be brought in. Freelance artists would be expected to supply their own kits, so it is important that they fully understand what the job entails. (A professional make-up kit is listed at the end of this chapter.)

The main focus in the studio make-up room is the professional make-up chair. This looks very much like the old barber's chair, which can be raised or lowered to the perfect height. Most studio make-up rooms do not have windows. They therefore have overhead strip lights as well as a well-lit mirror. The make-up chair always faces the mirror as the professional make-up artist has been trained to apply make-up using the mirror. The interviewer will also have total confidence in the person applying the make-up – it is after all the job of the make-up artist to know what looks correct on screen. Applying make-up through a mirror is much more critical than applying it directly onto a client. Most beauty therapists do not learn to work in this way.

Due to practicality and precise time schedules, skin care is not a consideration for the television make-up artist. Cleansers and toners may be used at the end of a programme if any of the guests or interviewers want the make-up removed.

Actor

Working on location may not always be the ideal situation in which to apply make-up. Depending on the budget and the level of production, the facilities will vary. It would be the responsibility of the freelance make-up artist to ensure that everything required is organized beforehand – a make-up supplier will not be readily available. Everything, down to the last detail, must be accounted for if the production is to run smoothly. The make-up to be applied on location should be worked out beforehand, taking into account factors such as temperature and climate which could affect the choice of products used.

REMEMBER

Products which create the desired effect in a studio may not be suitable on location.

On high budget films, a trailer would be available for use as a make-up room which would be kitted out with everything required for the production. Location chairs and mirrors are also available if necessary. Any freelance make-up artist working on location would have also worked in a studio and, therefore, would be capable of the organization required for a job such as this.

For detailed make-up effects, the application may take three to four hours. It is therefore not unusual for a make-up call to be around 5.00 a.m. The professional make-up artist is always the first there and the last to leave, having to prepare for the next day's shooting.

Model

This can be classed as one of the easiest areas of professional make-up to work in. The guidelines for preparing a salon client do not apply to the photographic or fashion model, as any skin care is the responsibility of the model, not the make-up artist. The main priority of the make-up artist is to check that the model's face is clear of any old make-up, especially mascara. If the model arrives from a former shoot with make-up on, it is the model's responsibility to remove it.

Models are usually chosen beforehand for their specific characteristics and style, which makes the make-up artist's job much easier when trying to create a certain look. For beauty shots, perfect features and no facial hair are essential. Ideally the skin will also be flawless, but this will depend on the level of model. Check the skin for dry patches around the nose, etc. If very obvious, an exfoliator may be required. It is unlikely that the skin would be excessively oily, as this would normally lead to spots. If a normal cleanser has been used to remove the make-up, remove any excess product with a toner. Some professional ranges provide a product which combines the cleanser and toner. This is ideal for the professional make-up artist as it is non-oily and will not leave a sticky residue on the surface of the skin.

Once the skin has been prepared, the eyebrows must be shaped to perfection. This means removing hair from any area above or below the brow. Most models are prepared to have the total eyebrow removed if that is the present fashion.

In preparing a male model for make-up, simply ensure that the skin is clean and free of any excess oil. Cotton wool should never be used as the fine particles will remain attached to any facial hair. Powder puffs are always used for applying powder and can be dampened and used to cleanse the skin as well.

Many of the top models apply their own make-up for the shows, but a make-up artist would always be on hand. Some flamboyant designers show collections for the catwalk which are more theatrical than they would ever sell in the stores. The make-up artist may then be asked to design a specific look. Depending on the number of models used, the make-up artist would work with one or possibly two assistants. The make-up artist would be freelance as shows are only put on at certain times in the year, but many designers use the same artist for every show. Because of the volume of work and the pressure under which they work, a hairdresser would also be employed at most of the big shows.

Most photographic studios have a basic make-up room or area which is kitted out with items such as heated rollers, an iron, hairspray, etc. However, not every studio would automatically supply all the items and it is worth enquiring beforehand. Make-up artists would always be required to bring their own kit as no make-up is supplied. It is unlikely, anyway, that they would be prepared to work with unfamiliar products. It is an advantage if the make-up artist is also able to style hair for session work, as it is less expensive for the client and may mean the difference as to whether an option is given or not.

—— PROFESSIONAL MAKE-UP KIT (BASIC CONTENTS) ——

Cleanser, toner, moisturizer

Exfoliator or strong astringent (for removing dry patches)

Foundation (light, medium and dark, in two textures)

Powder (translucent for all colour skins)

Eyeshadow selection (colours in contrasting tones)

Blusher selection (peach, pink, brown)

Lipstick selection (matt and gloss textures)

Eye pencils (black, grey, navy, brown)

Eyebrow pencils and shadows (taupe shades)

Lip pencils (various colours)

Eyeliner

Mascara

Frosted and dark loose powder

Eye drops

Eyelash curlers

Powder puffs

Tissues

Cotton buds

Make-up cape

Make-up brushes

Sewing kit

Water spray

Hair accessories (if required)

Straws (for models once lipstick is applied)

SUMMARY POINTS

- Moisturizer should be compatible with the foundation.
- Ensure all old make-up, especially mascara, is removed before you start work.
- Always check and shape the eyebrows *before* applying any make-up.
- Sit the salon client as straight as possible.

Questions

1 How would you recognize a moisturizer that is compatible with foundation?

2 How can oily skin be treated to stop the make-up disappearing?

3 How would you prepare a client for make-up who had excessively dry skin?

4 Why is it important to position the client vertically when applying make-up?

5 How would powder be applied to a male model?

2
Cosmetic products

KEY AREAS

At the end of this chapter you will know about:

• Cosmetic products in relation to a range of skin types and contexts

The range of products covered includes:

Sealer/anti-shine   Exfoliator
Moisturizer   Foundation
Powder   Eyeshadow/blusher
Eye pencil/lip pencil   Lipstick
Mascara   Eyebrow pencil/shadow
Eyeliner

The cosmetic industry, as we know it today, is so vast and competitive that it has forced a huge step forward in the development of cosmetic products. These now contain many sophisticated ingredients, moisturizing properties, fine particles of silk and UVA protection, which have replaced the fish scales and carbon black of the sixties. Today's products are so highly refined that they look and feel completely comfortable when applied to the skin. If make-up is applied well, it will conceal and enhance but never be obvious.

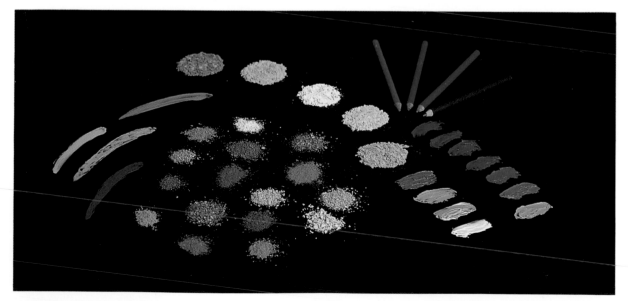

A selection of cosmetic products

Sealer/anti-shine

Because oily skin causes make-up to disappear quickly, many cosmetic companies now produce products which act as a barrier between the skin and the make-up, ensuring a much longer staying power. They work by forming a film over the surface of the skin – although the skin can then still produce oil, it cannot penetrate through to lift off the make-up. Many contain a silicone polymer ingredient which forms the seal, but each company has its own formulation. They can be applied over the entire face or just in areas that are particularly oily. Their textures vary, but they all do the same job.

The liquid forms dry completely, so it is important to check the oil and water content in the foundation being used over them. If the foundation has a high water content, the surface onto which it is applied should be slightly tacky to allow the movement needed for even blending. Other foundations with a higher oil content will already have enough movement for blending. It would be wise before deciding on the texture of the sealer to check the foundation first.

Solid textures of anti-shine are available. They also tend to dry completely, but it is usual to apply moisturizer under them first.

The cream forms of sealers can work in two ways. Either they are used in place of the moisturizer, or the sealer is allowed to absorb into the skin completely and the moisturizer applied over it.

Whichever texture you decide to use, this is an excellent product for dealing with the problems of oily skin.

Exfoliator

Excessively dry areas on the skin will be exaggerated once the foundation and the powder have been applied. They should always be removed before any application of make-up. Exfoliators are creams containing fine abrasive particles, which when worked over the top of a dry area will detach the small particles of dead skin. If, however, the dry area is sore or inflamed (for example at the sides of the nose due to a cold), it would not be advisable to use this particular product as it could irritate the skin further.

Shell Blast is the technical term used for the fine particles in these creams. They generally come from peach or walnut kernels which are ground very finely. Before the use of such natural ingredients, polyethylene was the synthetic substance employed.

Moisturizer

The biggest mistake a therapist is likely to make when applying make-up is the choice of moisturizer. The normal priority in beauty therapy is the skin. However, to apply make-up successfully, the therapist must put this priority on hold. Salon ranges of moisturizers are mostly treatment creams and do not work under make-up. Skin products provided by cosmetic companies are very different as they have to work with make-up. Skin care is a secondary factor for every large cosmetic company – they would certainly not sell products which were not compatible with the make-up.

The main use of moisturizer in professional make-up is to assist with the blending of foundation, especially ones which have a high water content. Sometimes the foundation can be applied directly onto the skin without the use of any moisturizer, which is why professional make-up can have a staying power of 12 hours. Professional make-up artists would generally carry only one moisturizer in their make-up kits – one which could be used on all skin types and with all foundations.

A compatible moisturizer will absorb into the skin completely, leaving no residue on the surface. If it is not totally absorbed it will affect the make-up in two ways. Firstly, because the skin must be completely dry to apply colour products perfectly, this would mean using more powder than necessary to dry out the foundation, having an unwanted 'ageing' effect on the client. Secondly, if not enough powder was used the foundation would remain sticky, causing the colour products to become patchy. Either way, the effect would be disastrous.

Moisturizer which is compatible with foundation absorbs totally into the skin, leaving no residue on the surface

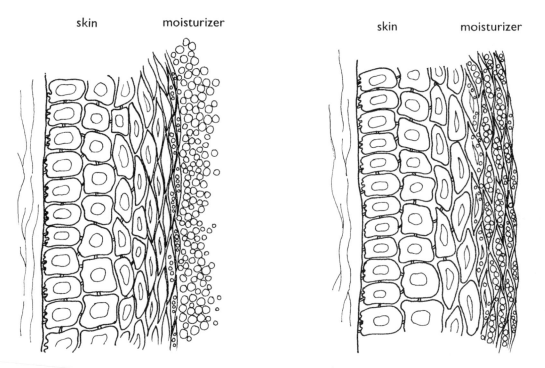

(a) *Moisturizer applied to the skin*   (b) *Moisturizer absorbed into the skin*

When working as a freelance make-up artist, the choice of moisturizer is entirely yours. This, however, is not so when a beauty therapist applies make-up. Here there is little choice in the matter unless you happen to own the salon that you are working in. Beauty therapists must use the products that the salon stocks, as they are also expected to retail these to the clients.

T I P

To test if a moisturizer is compatible with make-up application, take a small amount of the product and spread it thinly on the back of the hand. You are looking for any product which absorbs into the skin totally.

This test may take a few minutes to complete as each moisturizer absorbs at a different rate. Even if the product takes three or four minutes to absorb, it is still acceptable. In fact, different rates of absorption may be an advantage when deciding upon the right foundation. A foundation with a higher water content would be more compatible with a moisturizer which takes slightly longer to absorb. A foundation with a heavier texture, or one containing more oil, would work better over a moisturizer which absorbs more quickly.

REMEMBER

Choosing the right moisturizer makes all the difference to the staying power of the overall make-up.

Foundation

Foundation is used to even out the skin tone. It also creates the perfect canvas onto which the colour products are applied. Foundation is now available in many different textures as well as colours. The simplest breakdown of textures is to put them into categories of liquid, cream, solid and cake.

Liquid or cream?

Both liquid and cream foundations are made of a mixture of oil and water. Each cosmetic company has its own unique formulation which is protected as a very valuable company asset, especially if the product is one of the brand leaders. The original formulations of liquid and cream foundations had simple instructions to follow: cream was to be used on a dry skin, liquid was to be used on an oily skin. Today, this is not always followed, although it is still worth taking into consideration. The main difference stressed now is that cream gives better coverage and liquid gives a much more natural, see-through appearance. In making your decision, always choose the one which feels most comfortable on the client's skin.

Liquid foundation

Liquids now come in formulations that range from 100% water-based to 100% oil-based, as well as several variations in between. These variations of oil and water are designed for different skin types. Due to the FDA (Food and Drug Administration) in the United States, it is now law that any product sold must have a full listing of ingredients shown on the packaging, but this is not always helpful for the lay person.

Another very important characteristic of liquid foundation is that it can change colour on contact with the skin and may dry up to three shades darker. The colour change can be due to various factors, such as a higher oil content in the product itself, or the level of oil and acidity in the skin.

The simplest colours to choose from are light, medium and dark, in beige tones. If an identical colour match cannot be taken from one of these shades, they can be mixed together. Foundations with peach or pink pigments, which were very popular in the forties and fifties, produce an unnatural effect which is not acceptable for today's trends. The overall effect of liquid foundation is one that lets the natural skin tone glow through. It is ideally suited to the older skin as it does not accentuate age lines as much as the heavier textures. Because of the translucent effect of liquid foundation, it may be necessary to double the amount of product used in certain areas for extra coverage. Skin blemishes or high cheek colour do not warrant the use of a thicker foundation everywhere. If the liquid foundation is to be thickened in any particular area, a special technique is used to ensure that the extra product is not removed during the blending. (This technique will be explained in chapter 4.)

Cream foundation

With the obvious adaptability of liquid foundations, why do we need cream? There are, in fact, many advantages in choosing a cream, especially when first learning to apply foundation. The eager student will find a cream much easier to work with as the texture, being thicker, takes longer to dry. This gives the student more time to blend it to perfection. Cream foundations come in as many variations as liquid. They can vary in weight from a finely whipped soufflé to a much heavier greasy texture. The product can be tested on the back of the hand to establish the weight of the product.

There is very little colour change in a cream foundation as most do not dry completely until they are set with translucent powder. They are especially useful in photographic make-up when a flawless complexion is required. When applied correctly, cream foundation will not allow the skin tone to show through. However, by using less product and a little more pressure when blending, it can very easily duplicate the illusion of a liquid. The easiest colours to use are once again light, medium and dark, in beige tones – mixing two shades together if necessary.

Solid foundation

Solid foundation is the thickest texture and generally has a wax base. It is used mainly for theatrical products and has a colour range so extensive that it can incorporate more than a hundred shades. The theatrical name for solid foundation is greasepaint.

One main advantage in using solid foundation is that it does not have any colour change. This is because the product is so thick that the influence of the skin cannot affect it. Another advantage is its staying power. Solid foundation can vary in texture from a soft wax to a hard wax. The harder wax is dryer and therefore becomes waterproof, making it ideal for use in cosmetic camouflage products, and for swimming and other activities. In fact, if applied correctly (without moisturizer), it will remain on the skin until the client wishes to remove it. In some instances this may be as long as one week. The soft waxes have a greasy appearance, which means they will need more powder to set them. Many salon ranges still carry a range of wax products.

TIP . . . .

Use a damp sponge when applying solid foundation. This will thin the product, giving a much finer appearance.

. . . .

Cake foundation

Cake foundation, which was a development of Max Factor in the forties, is a powder and foundation all in one. The formulation is now very different from that of the original, as it has to be acceptable for today's market. Although it was formerly used mainly on oily skin, the product can now be used on any type of skin. The product is very convenient as it does not have to be set with translucent powder. It is generally applied with a damp sponge, although some companies do offer alternative methods. It is particularly successful in countries that have a hot, humid climate.

REMEMBER

When instructions are followed to the letter, all of the products present their own individual finish. However, with different blending techniques, combined with a variation in pressure when applying the product, any of the foundations can create the finish you wish to achieve.

Other varieties

Mousse

Another variation in texture is one that comes in an aerosol. It is called mousse and was a popular product in the eighties – possibly because the consumer was looking for something new. The finish of this foundation is very light, but it can be built up in the same way as liquid if extra coverage is required. The main points to be aware of are the dramatic colour change and the fact that the product has to be applied very quickly before its volume diminishes.

Tinted gels and moisturizers

Tinted gels and moisturizers are alternatives which can be used as a base for colour cosmetics. They would not, however, be classed as a foundation as they do not give any coverage to the skin. They should only be used on a perfectly clear complexion, to give the effect of a healthy skin. Dry skin should be well moisturized before applying these products, as they have a drying effect.

Concealers

Although concealers are still extensively used, they are, in fact, nothing more than a foundation. They generally come in two forms, solid and cream, and are really just a convenience product for those who do not have the expertise of professional techniques at their fingertips. Concealers only come in light shades and have no more than two variations in most ranges. The solid is a dry wax which appears in the form of a beige lipstick. The cream comes in a small tube rather like a mascara, but the end of the wand has a sponge applicator attached to it for easy application of the product onto the skin. The cream concealer has a high water content so that it dries within seconds of applying it to the skin. This allows more product to remain on the skin and not be removed during blending.

    If they have to be used, concealers are better applied on top of the foundation as the foundation itself may give the required amount of coverage. (Concealing techniques will be explained in chapter 4.) Worth considering is a new highlighter product by Yves Saint Laurent. It works well, yet is so fine in texture that it appears to disappear into the skin.

Foundation does not penetrate the skin when first applied, but acts as a barrier between the skin and the colour products (see diagram on page 26). It also protects the skin from damaging effects of the atmosphere and can contain a sun screen for added protection from the sun's rays. If foundation is applied correctly, it should feel completely comfortable on the skin – although the client who does not normally wear it may initially have to get used to it.

REMEMBER

Foundation must be removed completely at the end of the day, otherwise it will break down and small particles will be absorbed into the skin.

Foundation does not penetrate the skin when first applied and acts as a barrier between the skin and the colour products

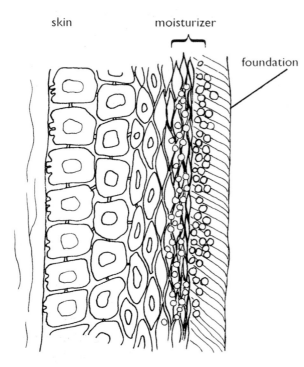

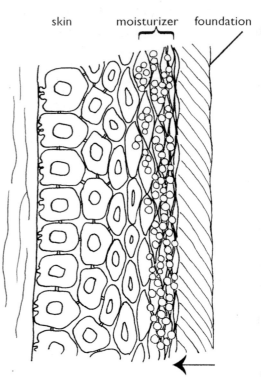

(a) *Moisturizer and foundation applied to the skin*

(b) *Moisturizer absorbs after two or three minutes, leaving the foundation on the surface*

Powder

All powders have a base of talc with various pigment colourings added. Those that appear slightly shiny have also had mica added. They come in two forms, solid and loose. Compact powders (solid) begin life in the same form as loose powders, but resin is added in the manufacturing process so that the powder particles will stick together. Sometimes, if too much resin has been added for the volume of powder used, it can be seen on the surface of the compact powder as a shiny film. This is, in fact, a faulty product as the shiny film has to be scraped off before any powder is released.

Loose powder should always be the first choice, whether it is to be used on a salon client or a model. Compact powder is mainly used for convenience and for re-touching throughout the day. It might occasionally be useful on a client with a much older, dryer skin, and only when a very thin foundation is required.

Powders are often described as translucent, but do not assume that all cosmetic companies use the term with the same meaning. It is, in fact, very difficult to find a powder that is totally translucent. Most powders contain some colour even when called translucent, and this should always be checked as it will alter the colour of the foundation. Application of a totally translucent powder is slightly different from one which contains colour (see chapter 4).

Powder is the most important of all the products when applying make-up. The amount needed will vary with the thickness of the foundation. Its main use is to absorb the oil content of the foundation, leaving the surface dry ready for the colour products. It will be clear at this point why the moisturizer should absorb totally into the skin; if it has not, too much powder will be needed to dry out the surface. Sometimes a soft sheen or glow may be required instead of a completely matt finish – on a black skin or an older skin, for example. Frosted powder can be dusted over the skin at the end of the make-up to produce this effect, although it should never be used to set the foundation.

Eyeshadow/blusher

I have grouped these together as they are basically the same product. Eyeshadows and blushers are used to emphasize the eyes and the shape of the face. Over past decades they have been used in various colours and styles to dictate the trend of the period.

Powder eyeshadows and blushers have a talc base, with colour pigment added and mica for a shiny finish. The original ingredient used to obtain the frosted look was fish scales. There is a vast difference in the texture of these shadows and blushers, which can affect the end result. Powder eyeshadows should not be too soft in texture, otherwise fine particles will fall onto the cheek bone during application. If a very dark shadow has been used, the particles may then be difficult to remove. Eyeshadows should also not be too hard, as then they are difficult to blend and may end up looking patchy.

TIP •

Always test any product before purchase, do not just rely on the visual impact. Take a small amount of product on the middle finger and gently blend it using the thumb. A good quality product should feel silky or creamy, which will blend beautifully when applied.

• •

Although eyeshadows and blushers are basically the same thing, there is a difference if they originate in the United States. The FDA have banned the use of natural pigment in all eyeshadows because they are used so close to the eyes. Natural pigment contains its own bacteria and if small particles get inside the eye they may cause problems. The natural pigment is therefore substituted with a synthetic equivalent called Carmine. This, unfortunately, is an expensive chemical and may result in the end product being a little more costly. Natural pigments are only used, however, to produce vibrant colours and will not be used in all shadows. The amount of colour pigment varies in all eyeshadows and blushers – it would be usual for products containing a higher proportion of pigment to cost more, but these would be easier to apply and worth it in the long term.

T●**P** . . . .

Products that contain less colour pigment are easily detected when checked on the back of the hand — the colour seen there will be very different from the colour in the palate.

. . . .

Cream blushers and eyeshadows are available, but mostly in the professional ranges. They are used either directly onto the skin if no foundation is worn (for example, on black skin or tanned skin) or between the foundation and the powder. They will not blend correctly if applied over powder. Their base is wax with colour pigment added, much the same as the wax foundations, and their textures vary. They were most popular in the sixties when cosmetic products were still quite basic, but they are still commonly used, particularly in theatrical make-up.

Liquid blusher is also available. It comes in the same form as a liquid foundation, but is coloured. The texture is extremely fine and is applied following the same guidelines as for cream.

Choosing which texture to use depends on the overall effect you want to create. Sometimes two textures can be used together. For example, if the colour of the blusher fades much more quickly than the other cosmetics the client is wearing, cream blusher should be applied before the powder and powder blusher over it. This method will achieve a more lasting effect.

Eye pencil/lip pencil

The only difference between eye pencils and lip pencils is their colour. As for all cosmetic preparations, their textures and quality differ enormously. The ideal pencil, whether for eyes or lips, should be one that applies easily. If the texture is too hard, the pressure used may distort the skin and produce very little colour. If the pencil is too soft, it could cause creasing around the eyes and bleeding around the mouth. The product is again wax based, varying from a hard to a soft texture.

T●**P** . . . .

If the texture of the pencil you already have is too soft, it can be placed in the refrigerator to stiffen it slightly rather than discard it. Pencils which are a little too hard can be rotated in a tissue between the ends of the fingers. The friction created by this motion softens the end of the pencil, making it easier to use, particularly around the eye area.

. . . .

The amount of pigment in pencils varies, as in the other colour cosmetic products. It is advisable to check the colour and texture of the pencil on the back of the hand before purchasing it.

Lipstick

Lipsticks over the years have changed their colour and texture to coincide with fashion looks. The last 50 years of style have given us a wide range of textures to use, from dry matt textures to soft glossies. Lipstick has a base of wax containing colour pigment. Textures vary as does the density of the pigment – test the lipstick (as with all the other products) on the back of the hand. The final choice of lipstick will depend on the finished effect required. However, there are several other points to be taken into consideration first.

POINTS TO NOTE

- A slightly softer texture of lipstick may be better suited to the more mature skin, whereas the more popular style may be the matt finish.
- Different lipstick textures possess different staying powers. Softer textures will disappear more quickly, particularly if the client generates a lot of body heat.
- Frosted lipsticks have a slightly longer staying power because the mica which creates the frost makes them slightly dryer.
- The harder, dry matt textures will have the longest staying power, but are not always suited to the mature skin.

The texture should also be considered carefully if a client complains of the lipstick bleeding. This generally occurs where the client produces a lot of body heat, or uses a texture of lipstick which is too soft. Most lipsticks come in stick form, but soft textures may be in pots. It would not be appropriate to produce these textures in stick form as they would break too easily.

Mascara

All mascaras are water resistant but only a few are still waterproof. The wide range of colours fashionable in the seventies has now died out to some extent, but who can predict what will be fashionable in the future?

Mascaras come in two forms, cake and cream. Cream is the most widely used texture. It comes in a tube which has a wand for easy application. Cake mascara had its heyday in the fifties. The block was wet by spitting on it, which, strangely enough, worked better than water. This is, however, unacceptable for today's hygiene-conscious therapists.

The most widely used colours in mascara are black and brown. A few years ago the cosmetic companies seemed to cash in on the latest fashion of clear mascara. It was only after millions of products were sold that most women realized this did not work at all unless they had been blessed with thick, long, dark eyelashes.

Mascara has a wax base containing a percentage of water. A full list of ingredients is provided at the end of this chapter.

Eyebrow pencil/shadow

Eyebrows create our facial expression as well as being the framework for the eyes. A perfectly shaped eyebrow should need little else than a light comb to remove excess foundation and powder which may be attached to the hair. Where necessary, however, there are two products which can be used to enhance eyebrow shape: eyebrow pencils and shadows.

Eyebrow pencils come in various colours, the most versatile being taupe (grey/brown). Their texture may be slightly firmer than the eye pencil, but the area on which they are used (the brow bone) is also firmer.

Eyebrow shadows also have a harder texture than normal shadows, but again they are applied onto a much firmer surface. The colour selection is much wider than for pencils and they are more easily available.

In some cases a better effect is achieved when the two products are used together.

Eyeliner

During the sixties, few women would have been seen without eyeliner. It is a product that comes in and out of fashion, yet the finish it creates to any professional make-up is superb. It is available in cake, liquid, and the newest form which resembles a type of felt pen. The most popular colour is, of course, black. Whatever the size or shape of the eyes, eyeliner will undoubtedly make them appear larger. It can be used on any age or style of make-up, especially to add a hint of glamour.

——— MAKE-UP INGREDIENTS ———

POWDER
Base
Talc
Preservatives
Methylparaben
Propylparaben
Sodium dehydroacetate

LIPSTICK
Wax for stick structure
Beeswax
Candelilla wax
Ozokerite
Carnauba
Paraffin
Skin conditioning agents
Mineral oil
Isopropyl myristate
Lanolin oil
Wheat germ glycerides
Corn oil
Acetylated lanolin alcohol

Anti-oxidant
Propylene glycol + RHA + propyl gallate + citric acid
Pigment solvent
Castor oil
Pigments
Titanium dioxide
D&C red 6 barium lake
D&C red 7 calcium lake
D&C red 27 aluminium lake
D&C yellow 5 aluminium lake
D&C yellow 6 aluminium lake
D&C blue 1 aluminium lake
Iron oxides
Manganese violet
Pearl agents
Mica
Bismuth oxychloride

MASCARA
Base
Water
Stearic acid
Beeswax
PVP
Oxtyldodecanol
Carnauba
Viscosity control agent
Butylene glycol
pH adjuster
Triethanolamine
Emulsifying agent
Sorbitan sesquioleate
Preservatives
Methylparaben
Propylparaben
Pigments
Chromium hydroxide
Titanium dioxide
Iron oxides

SUMMARY POINTS

- Make the products work for you. Foundations can always be adapted by varying the amount of product and the pressure used.
- Never buy any cosmetic product without testing it first — it only takes a minute!

Questions

1 For what purpose do we use foundation?

2 Why do we use powder?

3 Why do we wear blusher?

4 What causes lipstick to bleed?

5 How would you find the right foundation colour?

3
Tools of the trade

As for any profession, the right tools are an important factor in making the job easier and in creating a professional result. There are many accessories available to assist in make-up application, as well as a large selection of brushes. The most important aspect in choosing your tools is finding the right size and shape for the area you are working on. This may differ for each individual, which is why professional make-up brushes have no guidelines for their particular use. Shape and size may vary according to personal preference – the essential characteristic is that the application can be done with ease and finished to perfection.

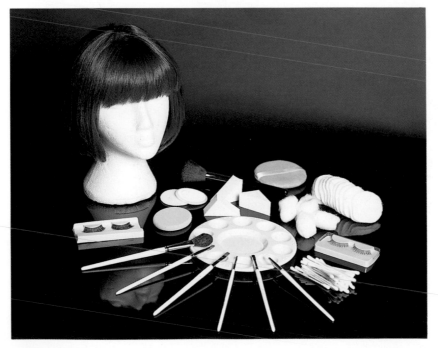

A selection of make-up tools

Brushes

There is a big difference in the price and quality of make-up brushes available today. Most of the cheaper brushes are made of pony hair and are machine manufactured in the Far East. The best brushes are made of sable hair and are handmade. If looked after, they will last a lifetime. They are sold individually so that, although they are more expensive than their cheaper counterparts, a set can be built up over a period of time. A good selection of professional brushes can cost in the region of £100.

The range of shapes and sizes is huge, but the easiest way to select them is to go by the head shape. The three different styles are flat top, round top or hovis, filbert or point. They are sized in fractions of inches which can vary from one-eighth to two inches. The volume of hair within each brush can also change its style. There are many specialized brushes for particular uses, but the final choice is down to the individual – use the one that you feel most comfortable with.

The metal section which attaches the hair to the handle is called a ferrule. In some of the smaller brushes this will be completely circular, but in the larger ones it will be nipped to change the shape of the hair.

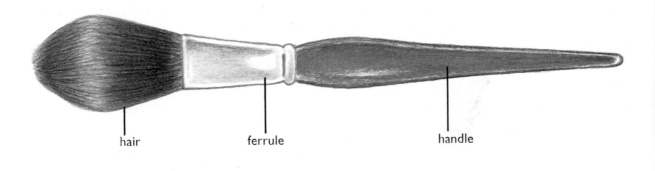

hair   ferrule   handle

A standard make-up brush

Powder brush

This is the largest of all the brushes and is generally made of pony hair. To use sable for this particular brush would be far too expensive and, in fact, too soft to give the brush the correct pressure. The correct application for powder is with the powder puff, but the professional kit should always include a powder brush as well. It is used to add finishing touches, or possibly for any work on the body. The powder brush will add a light film of powder, but will not absorb the oil content of the foundation too much to make it completely dry.

The powder brush can be used at the end of a make-up to add extra colour. If, for example, the foundation appears a little too pale, colour can be added with the powder brush and a slightly darker powder. If a slightly frosted look is required by either the client or the model (sometimes older clients prefer this look), frosted powder can be lightly dusted over the entire face at the end of the make-up.

The hair of the powder brush should be slightly domed at the end. If the brush has been machine manufactured, there will be sharp lines where the hair has been chopped. This creates a much stiffer pressure to the end of the hair and can lead to patchy application of the powder. The hard edge may also interfere with the foundation. It is important to check for this ridge before purchasing large brushes. The final third of the hair should be shaped, tapering virtually to a point.

Blusher brush

The blusher brush is the same shape as the powder brush, therefore all of the aforementioned points apply. Only the overall size is different. The blusher brush should be approximately 25 mm (one inch) across the top of the ferrule.

The hair should not be much wider than 25 mm (one inch) as it will double in size (with the pressure) when it touches the cheek bone. Note that 50 mm (two inches) is about the average width between the top and bottom of the cheek bone. There are many larger blusher brushes available, but these give less control over the placement of the colour.

Contour brush

Professional contour brushes are used today mainly for character and period make-up. They are hovis-shaped, flat, sable brushes which are available in various sizes. Since the natural looks of the eighties, contouring in everyday make-up has become unfashionable.

Machine-manufactured brush sets usually contain a rather odd-shaped, short, flat brush, labelled 'contour' on its handle. The pressure from this brush would create a strong solid line down the side of the face and is unsuitable for the natural effects required in current make-up styles.

Eyeshadow brush

Eyeshadow brushes vary in the shape and size of the head (flat, hovis and filbert). The choice of shape and size is left to each individual as there are no guidelines given on the handle. The pressure of each brush will vary with its size and shape. The correct pressure is very important to the end result, so the heads should always be checked when deciding which brush to use in a particular area on the face. If the ferrule is round, it will contain more hair and the pressure of the brush will be lighter. If the ferrule is flat then the pressure will be a lot firmer.

Sable is the main type of hair used in these brushes, with goat hair substituted in the less expensive ones. Different qualities of cosmetics require the use of different brushes. This will enable the make-up artist to vary the finished effect.

Lip brush

The lip brush is, in fact, the same as the eyeshadow brush. The small-sized, sable brushes give the correct pressure for applying lipstick. The best shape to use when learning is the flat top (see chapter 4), although many established make-up artists do prefer the filbert. The one-eighth inch is the best size for the harder wax lipsticks. For the slightly softer textures, the size can be anything between one-eighth and three-sixteenths.

Eyebrow brush

There are a selection of brushes for the eyebrows. The angled eyebrow brush is one of the few brushes which has to be made of nylon to work effectively. It is used to apply eyebrow shadow, when darkening blonde eyebrow hair for example. The effect is sometimes much softer than the eyebrow pencil. However, even if you do use a pencil, the angled eyebrow brush can still be used to soften any strong lines. This brush is an essential part of any professional brush kit.

The brush and comb or small toothbrush style is made of nylon or boar hair. It is a useful brush for combing the eyelashes, as well as the eyebrow hair, if there is a build up of powder or foundation.

The one other alternative resembles a mascara wand. This again can be used to comb the eyelashes as well as the eyebrows. For example, if the eyelashes have become clogged together with mascara, this brush will separate them – but make sure it is then free of mascara before using it on the eyebrows.

The choice between these three brushes is down to the individual make-up artist. All three would be very useful to have and, because they are made of synthetic fibres, are fairly inexpensive.

Eyeliner brush

There is only one style of eyeliner brush, used for the application of cake eyeliner. The other two eyeliner products come with their own applicator. Although these are the smallest of all the brushes, they are available in different sizes.

The ferrule on the eyeliner brush should be round and the hair will be either sable or nylon. The pony or squirrel hair used in machine-made kits retains no pressure at all and will collapse on contact with the skin. Soft nylon will keep its shape and pressure better than any other, even the sable one.

Professional make-up suppliers generally carry the sable liner brush, but a good art shop can supply the equivalent in nylon and has several size variations. As eyeliner is applied in different thicknesses (on each person, as well as to create different effects), a comprehensive brush collection should always have two or three different sizes in it.

Sponge-tipped applicators

Sponge-tipped applicators are used in the application of eyeshadows. The choice of whether to use a sponge tip in preference to a brush is up to the individual artist. There are, however, many advantages in using a sponge tip, particularly when applying dark shadows. For example, when the shadow is taken onto the foam pad it can be worked on the back of the hand before it is transferred to the eyelid. This motion grinds the small particles of shadow into the pad so that fewer particles will fall below the eye on application. Any colour applied with the sponge-tipped applicator will also show its depth immediately. Up to 50% of the colour can be lost if eyeshadow is applied with a brush. In addition, the applicator has two distinct sides, so the shadow can be applied with one and blended with the other.

Sponge tips come in different shapes; round, square and pointed. My particular preference is for the square type as it does not have a hard seam around it where the foam has been heat sealed. The edge of the square sponge can therefore be used without scratching the delicate skin around the eye area. Foam is the material used for the pad of the sponge tip, but the texture varies. Brushed foam has a softer feel and, in fact, allows the shadow to blend more successfully.

Application sponges (for foundation)

There are several variations of applicators which can be used to apply foundation. They are explained in detail in chapter 4. Each one has its advantages when used in conjunction with the different textures of foundation, but the final choice is down to the individual artist.

Powder puffs

Powder puffs come in various sizes. Their main use is for the application of loose powder, particularly on males as cotton wool attaches itself to facial hair.

The large ones, which are approximately 100 mm (four inches) across, have a satin band across one side. Professional make-up artists use this band over their small finger so that the puff can be used as a pad between the back of the hand and the area on which they are working. This is important for hygiene and is also an advantage when working with heavy bases, such as in theatrical make-up. Otherwise, if the make-up artist has warm hands, an imprint will be left in the foundation or the foundation may be lifted off when the hand is removed.

The new style is much smaller, approximately 63 mm (two and a half inches) across. Some of this type have a satin pouch covering half of one side. Make-up artists who have large hands sometimes use the pouch over the ends of their fingers, which gives them more control in difficult areas.

Eyelash curlers

Not all make-up artists feel comfortable using eyelash curlers. However, it is an item which should be part of your kit as models often like to use eyelash curlers themselves. They do make a considerable difference on many people, particularly if the eyelashes are very straight. I personally do not recommend them as they can break the eyelash hairs or even pull them out.

Tweezers

Tweezers are an essential part of any make-up kit. They are available in three styles; pointed, straight and slanted. Always make sure that the tweezers are able to extract the hair and bulb completely without cutting it. Tweezers should be cleaned (or sterilized for beauty therapists) after each use with 90° proof alcohol. Quite often the skin will bleed if the eyebrow hair is very thick – hygiene, therefore, must be a priority.

Pencil sharpener

The most popular sharpeners for a make-up kit have two different sized holes to accommodate any size of pencil. When sharpening pencils, always remember to round off the point. This is especially important for eye pencils. If they are too pointed, they will drag the skin around the eye area. They could also be dangerous this close to the eye. Keep your pencil sharpener clean with 90° proof alcohol and sharpen the pencils between each use when working on clients.

Tissues

There is no mystery to using tissues, but they are essential in any make-up application. Do not scrub or wipe the face with a tissue, blot it. The tissue should be pressed against the skin then lifted off. This motion is called stippling and will be explained in chapter 4.

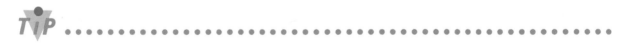

To blot excess oil from the foundation before applying powder, cotton wool can be placed inside the tissue to create a small pad. This will work much better than the tissue on its own as the cotton wool inside will provide a firmer surface. Tissues supplemented in this way can also be dampened and used to lift off excess powder, and can be used around the neckline to protect clothing.

Cotton buds

The modern make-up artist would be lost without cotton buds. They are very useful in keeping the eye make-up tidy. They are used to clean the eye corners, to blend shadow and to correct errors. For example, if mascara has been smudged accidentally onto the skin, it is vital to act quickly before the mascara dries. Point the cotton tip directly onto the skin and turn it quickly from side to side between the thumb and the first finger. If the mascara has not been allowed to dry, it will lift off immediately. A cotton bud can also be used to correct the lip line if a mistake has been made, without having to start again.

There are many more tools and variations of brush style that could be mentioned, but the ones covered here are the most important to any artist's kit. The choice of any of them is finally down to individual preference. Whichever you decide to use, make sure you keep them meticulously clean. Always let your brushes dry naturally – the tighter the hair when wet, the better the shape when dry. Caring for your make-up brushes will keep them in good condition and help them to retain their shape. They will then last you a lifetime.

SUMMARY POINTS

- Always let brushes dry naturally – the tighter the hair when wet, the better the shape when dry.
- Invest in good brushes, and care for them – they will last you a lifetime.

Questions

1 How can eyeshadows retain their intensity when applied to the skin?

2 In professional make-up brushes, the shape of the hair varies depending on what the brush is used for. Name the different styles available.

3 What is the best way to clean brushes which have been used to apply a product which contains wax or oil?

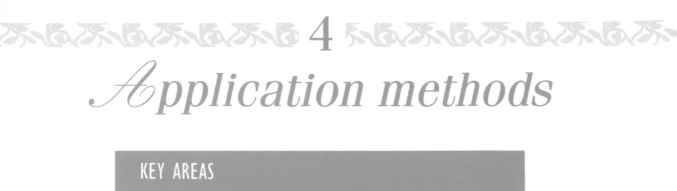

4
Application methods

KEY AREAS

By the end of this chapter you will be able to:

- Select and agree make-up with the client
- Apply make-up using efficient techniques
- Apply make-up in the correct sequence
- Apply strip and single lashes, and give the appropriate aftercare

All make-up artists will have favourite methods for applying make-up. If you are not yet completely comfortable with the techniques you are using, then this book will help you decide. You can try all the methods before making your final decision, but the ones you do choose should be comfortable for both you and your client.

REMEMBER

Pressure is the vital factor in applying today's cosmetics.

Cleanser

Deep cleansing treatment is not advisable before any make-up application – it could load the skin with too many creams which would cause the make-up to slide off if not removed thoroughly. A basic cleansing is all that is required before make-up is applied. This will remove any superficial dirt which has settled on the surface of the skin. It is not the job of the make-up artist to look after the skin (see chapter 1). Skin care is not a priority here, the make-up is. I will therefore mention cleansing only briefly – there are many excellent beauty therapy books available if further detail is required.

If make-up is applied in a salon situation, there will be many different types of cleansers available. A basic cleanser is adequate before make-up. Using one that is too heavy may leave residue on the surface of the skin and therefore affect the end result of the make-up.

For cleansing the face, you should ideally be positioned behind the client. This is the usual routine when working in a salon, but may not be possible outside the salon situation. The cleanser is applied to the skin with damp cotton wool. (Eye make-up must be removed first with a non-oily eye make-up remover.) Gentle circular movements should be used in an upward motion. If, however, you have to work from a front position, the cleansing movements should be directed towards the centre of the face.

Toner

Toners are used to remove excess cleanser which has been left on the surface of the skin. It is vital that no cleanser remains on the skin, otherwise this will create problems when the cosmetics are applied. Some toners are stronger and may be called astringents or clarifying lotions. The variation is due to the different skin types. Excessively oily skin will require a toner which has a slightly higher alcohol content.

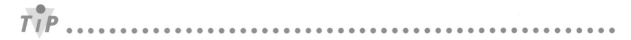

TIP

Some of the professional skin care companies have produced a cleanser and toner in one. This is ideal for any make-up artist as it can be used throughout the make-up application on any area that needs correcting, without leaving a greasy film. I use one from an Italian company called DIBI.

Toner is applied in the same way as the cleanser, but the cotton wool should not be too damp – otherwise it will weaken the strength of the product and will not remove all of the cleanser.

Moisturizer

Again, the most effective position for applying moisturizer is from behind. The client will ideally be seated on a facial couch which can be adjusted to the correct height. The moisturizer is then applied to the skin using the fingers, starting from the chin and working upwards. Moisturizers used as part of a salon treatment would differ from those used under make-up.

Professional make-up artists are unable to follow this procedure as their studio chairs do not adjust sufficiently to allow them to operate from behind. Studio chairs do, however, adjust in height to make it more comfortable for the make-up artist. Location chairs have a fixed height so that any application of product must be carried out from the side or front position. Although moisturizers may still be applied using the fingers, the side or front position can make this quite awkward. An alternative is to apply the moisturizer with a sponge. The best sponge to use would be a wedge. It is important to use a sponge that is dry as damp sponges tend to absorb a certain amount of the moisturizer.

The product should be blended over the entire face, including the eyelids and lips. It should also be taken down the neck, even if the foundation is not taken that far down.

Foundation

There are various different methods of applying foundation, all of which are totally acceptable in professional make-up. Some methods do, however, work better with particular textures of foundation.

TiP . . . .

Through practise, the time taken to apply the foundation will get shorter — until then always apply foundation section by section, as some foundations dry very quickly and could become patchy.

. . . .

Blending with fingers

Although blending with fingers is not a readily accepted method of application for salon make-up, some well-established make-up artists will use no other method. In certain areas of professional make-up it may be essential that the fingers are used in order for the product to blend correctly. One such area is theatrical make-up. Wax foundations blend better when applied with the fingers as the warmth from them helps to soften the wax. Wax products will not dry until they are set with powder and can therefore be dotted all over the face and then blended. They do not have to be worked section by section like some of the other products. The pads of the last two index fingers are usually the most comfortable to use.

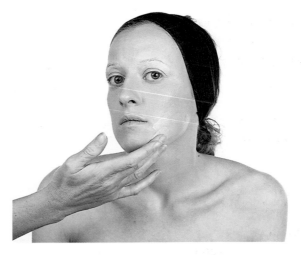

Blending foundation with the fingers. The base is being applied for Elizabeth I *character make-up*

Damp sponge method

There are various shapes and sizes of sponges that can be used damp – most of them are round or oval. Any of the foundation textures can be applied with a damp sponge and, because the foundation is blended downwards, the effect can be quite sheer. If any area needs extra coverage, the foundation is stippled over that particular area. Stippling is a rolling motion where the pressure starts at one side of the sponge and is carefully moved through to the other (imagine the old Victorian ink blotter). The damp sponge can be dipped directly into the liquid foundation and worked from the back of the hand onto the face.

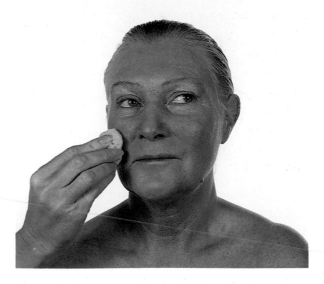

Blending foundation with a damp sponge.

Wedge sponge method

The wedge was designed in the seventies as an alternative to the damp sponge. The original wedge was made of 100% latex rubber, although there have since been many variations produced. Wedge sponges do not absorb water.

The wedge can be used to apply all textures of foundation, but for liquid and cream it is advisable to use a small brush to dot the product onto the skin first. Because liquid and cream foundations can change colour on contact with the skin, they should be applied as quickly as possible and in sections. This will avoid the foundation going patchy during the application.

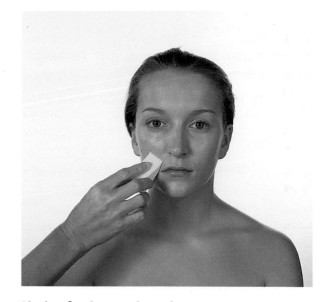

Blending foundation with a wedge sponge

REMEMBER

A very light pressure is needed when using a wedge to blend, otherwise the product may be lifted back off the skin during the application.

The shape of the wedge gives it a unique quality which no other applicator possesses. The angles of the wedge each have a different pressure which can alter the finished effect of the foundation.

The lightest angle of the wedge is also useful for blending foundation into corners, such as the side of the nose or the corner of the eye. As long as the wedge is dry, it can be used throughout the make-up application. For example, if eyeshadow has fallen onto the cheek bone or if the blusher colour has been applied too heavily, the wedge can be used to remove it. The wedge cannot be used to build up the foundation if extra coverage is needed. It may therefore be necessary to combine this with another method.

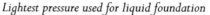

Lightest pressure used for liquid foundation

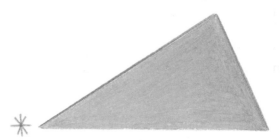

Medium pressure used for cream foundation or blending the edges of liquid foundation

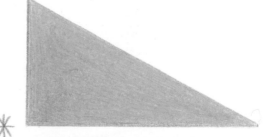

Heaviest pressure for rubbing out colour or base

Painting method

This method is still fairly new to the industry, but is certainly the best when a flawless finish is required. The technique is ideal for photographic make-up or for the client who needs a little extra coverage.

The painting method can be used with any of the textures of foundation. It is important that the painting brush is kept as dry as possible throughout the application, even if the brush has to be rubbed several times into a tissue. Because of this, liquid or cream foundation should be dotted onto the skin first with a smaller brush.

Avoid building up too much foundation as it could lead to the product streaking. The painting brush can be moved in any direction, even against the facial hair. In fact, the more directions the brush is moved in, the better the result. Slightly more pressure should be applied to the brush initially so that the foundation is moved over the entire area. A lighter pressure should be used to finish off the blending – to remove any streaks in the base. As the painting brush is made of sable (sable does not hold water), it can be washed between each use.

Flat sponge method

Many cosmetic companies supply round, flat sponges with their solid foundations. They are made of a percentage of latex and can be used either wet or dry. They can be used to apply any of the foundation textures. If dampened first, these sponges will thin out the texture of the foundation being applied, which may be required for some make-up styles.

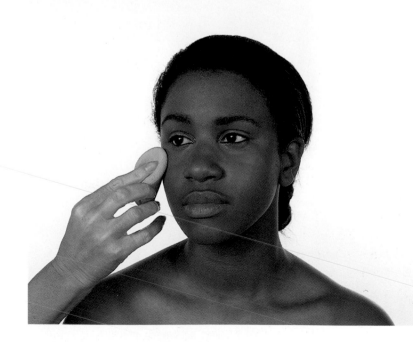

Blending foundation with a flat sponge

Powder

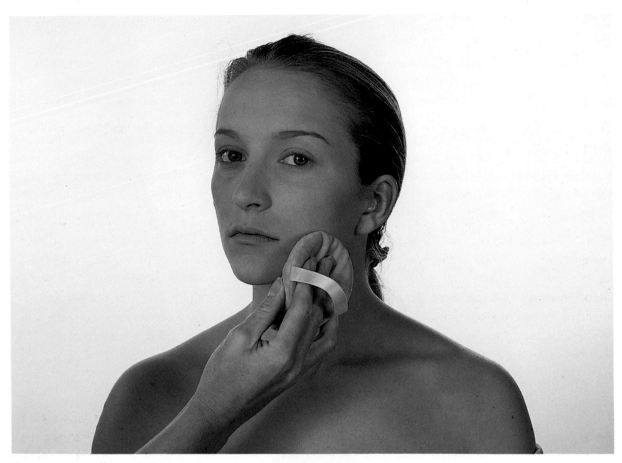

Using a powder puff to apply loose powder

REMEMBER

Powder is used to dry out the surface onto which the colour is to be applied. This will include any stickiness from the skin and excess moisturizer, as well as the oil content of the foundation. The preparation beforehand and use of a compatible moisturizer are therefore important factors in applying the correct amount of powder.

TIP

The best method of applying powder professionally is with a powder puff. Because of hygiene considerations, round cottonwool pads would be the disposable alternative in a salon situation. If cottonwool pads are used, three would give a similar thickness to the puff — using one would produce an uneven pressure.

The powder is applied by stippling (blotting) it onto the foundation. Care should be taken when applying powder – too much pressure would smudge the foundation and wiping the powder on would not absorb the oil content sufficiently. Water-based foundations require less powder to dry them out, while oil-based products will require more.

T¡P ....

The amount of powder contained on the pad should always be checked on the back of the hand, never applied directly onto the skin.

Because of their lack of pigment, true translucent powders may give a chalky effect to the skin if not applied correctly. This type of powder should be applied a little at a time, each layer being totally absorbed before the next is applied, to prevent a build up of product. Powders should also be applied section by section, concentrating on one area until it is completely dry before moving onto the next. The finished area can be checked with the back of the hand to be sure that it is completely dry.

T¡P ....

A little excess powder should be left on the surface of the skin throughout the rest of the make-up application. It will absorb quickly into the foundation due to the amount of body heat generated and, in the long run, will give a longer staying power to the total make-up. All colour products will blend more easily if the surface onto which they are applied is completely dry.

The powder brush is used for applying tinted or frosted powders at the end of the make-up. The tip of the powder brush should be dipped into the powder and transferred into the lid of the powder pot. Powder should never be transferred directly onto the skin as 80% will be deposited on the area that is touched, resulting in a patchy finish. When the powder is deposited into the lid, the brush should be moved quickly in a clockwise direction. Before the brush touches the skin, check that there are no solid particles remaining. This application can be repeated several times if a colour change (lighter or darker) is required – for example, if the foundation was not colour matched correctly at the beginning.

Although the cosmetic companies also produce compact powder, this is used only occasionally in professional make-up. Examples are if an extremely light finish is required, or on a much older client when a very thin layer of foundation has been used. Its application is the same as for loose powder.

Eyebrow shaping

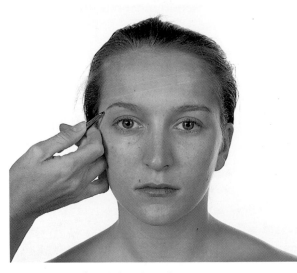

Removing hair from below the eyebrow

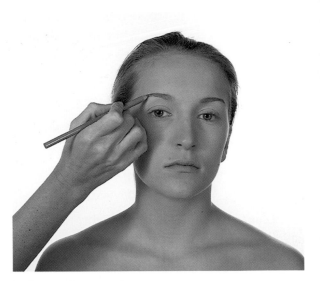

Applying eyebrow pencil

Shaping eyebrows has always been a controversial issue within the beauty industry. The basic guidelines for shaping are quite specific – hair should only be removed from the underside of the brow and the basic shape should never be altered. These are suitable ground rules for the novice. With experience, however, they will be expanded to enable the therapist to deal confidently with any unforeseen variation. This will include removing hair from any area above or below the natural line, as necessary.

Eyebrows can be made to appear fatter or thinner, or even removed altogether if fashion dictates this. Little attention was paid to the eyebrows in the eighties, when it was fashionable to let them take their natural shape. Now the nineties has established itself, there is renewed emphasis on the perfect eyebrow. However, style or fashion should never dictate a limit to the professional make-up artist's ability.

Initially, the best guideline to follow is the brow bone. As seen in the diagram overleaf, a line is drawn from the centre point at where the eyebrow begins, up to its highest point and down again to its tail end. This line will establish the arch over the highest point of the brow bone. It is best drawn with eyebrow pencil, not shadow, and it is important that the line drawn is continuous, without the pencil leaving the skin. Once this initial line has been drawn, it can be gradually thickened on either side (mainly on the first section) to create the desired effect. The tail end of the eyebrow should become narrower as it gently slopes down towards the temple.

TIP •

Two different colours of eyebrow pencil will give a much more natural effect.

• •

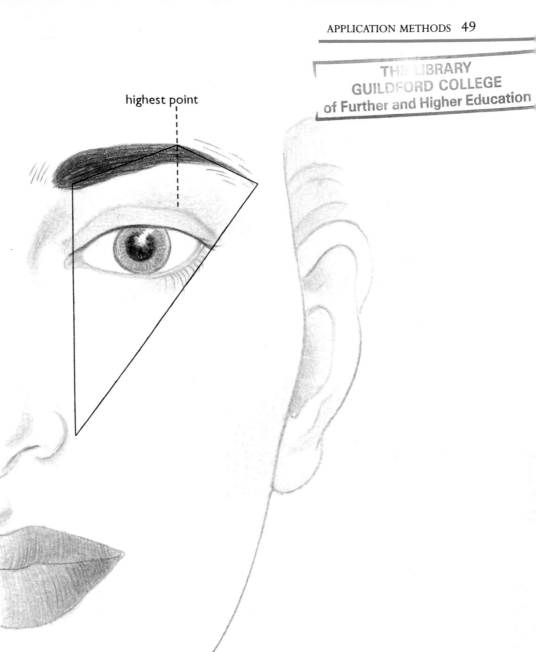

highest point

Guidelines to creating the perfect eyebrow. Remove any hairs outside the main edge

Eyebrow shadow can be used if the hair of the eyebrow is blonde or if a much softer effect is required. The shadow should be applied in small strokes, using slightly more pressure at the beginning of the hair so that the colour there appears slightly darker, making it look more natural. If it is necessary to apply the shadow directly onto the skin, use the same small strokes. In some cases, a pencil may be used on the skin for the last section; to create a sharper finish.

Eyeshadow

Eyeshadow can be applied by using either a sponge-tipped applicator or various sizes of eyeshadow brush.

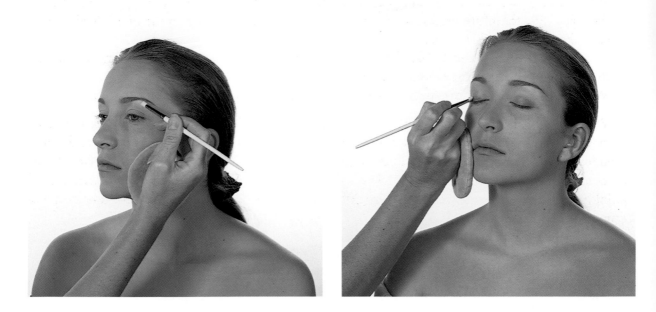

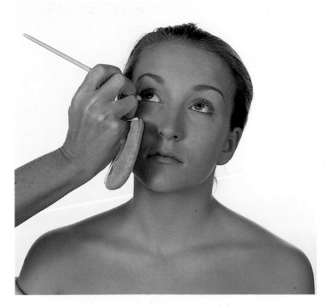

Applying eye-shadow. A puff is used to protect the area being worked on

POINTS TO NOTE

- When blending, a variation in pressure will produce a perfectly faded edge of colour, as well as creating a different depth of colour.
- When the eyeshadow first touches the skin, 80% of the colour is immediately deposited in that area. It is therefore important to make sure that the area on which the brush is placed can take this amount of colour.
- If the same colour is used to blend away the shadow's edge, remove some first on the back of the hand and reload from there.
- When applying eyeshadow to the older client, neutral colours are most successful.

Vibrant colours are definitely out. The look of the nineties is achieved by using a variation in techniques rather than a variation in colour. For example, by using two muted shades and clever blending, a beautiful, sophisticated look can be easily created. Definite colour on the face should be confined to the lips and the cheeks. The fashion industry has expanded the boundaries of colour that we wear in our clothes, which is why we cannot now indulge with the same scope in our cosmetics.

Blusher

There are two reasons why we wear blusher; to add colour and to give shape. When applying blusher, the area to concentrate on is therefore the cheek bone. When working on models who have naturally prominent cheek bones, applying blusher is just a matter of colouring the prominent area. This, however, is not the case for most clients.

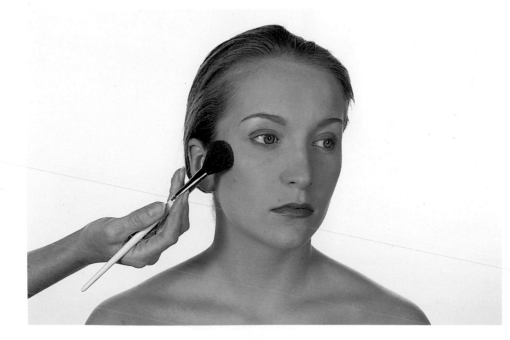

Study the guidelines below before applying any colour. They apply to any face shape. The blusher and lipstick should always come from the same colour group. If only one blusher colour is to be used, it should be applied more heavily on the baseline and more lightly on the top edge nearest to the eye.

The baseline should be found using the handle of one of the smaller brushes. Holding the brush in position, take an imaginary line from the corner of the mouth to the centre of the ear. On most people the top of the bulb at the front of the ear will run parallel with the cheek bone – this is the line to work from.

The guidelines for the baseline are the same on everyone. If the cheek bone is not obvious, leave the handle in position against the face while applying the colour. When the brush is loaded with colour, it should touch the face at the hairline first and then be moved slowly from left to right along the baseline.

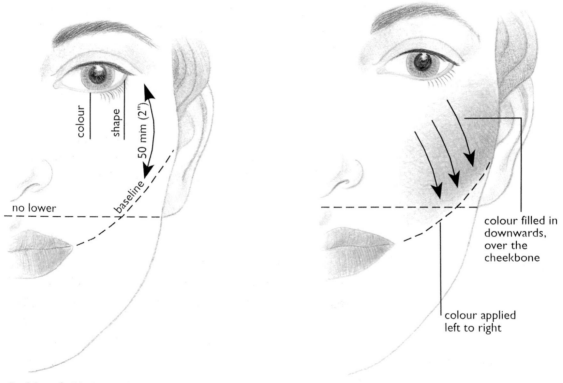

Guidelines for blusher application   Application of blusher over the cheek bone

REMEMBER

The first point of the face touched will have 80% of the colour unloaded on it. The centre of the face cannot take that amount of colour, the hairline can.

Repeat if necessary. Once the baseline has been established, the colour can be applied carefully over the cheek bone (see above diagram). Build up the colour until the desired effect is created.

An alternative to this method, which gives a darker effect at the base, is to use two colours. The darker colour is used under the bone and the lighter one is used over the bone. The guidelines, however, are still the same.

REMEMBER

Make-up today should be part of the face. (The old guidelines for blusher were to work against the shape, not with it.) The depth of colour and how far the colour is brought into the centre of the face will alter the shape.

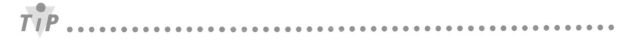

TIP

Sometimes the edge on the top side of the blusher may have been applied too heavily. If this has happened it is very easy to correct. First try wiping it away with a dry wedge or, alternatively, blend some translucent powder over the line. Use the two methods together if necessary. If the blusher has emphasized any skin problems, remove it with a clean, dry wedge. Then rebuild the colour using alternate layers of powder and blusher.

The wide range of blusher colours available today has replaced the use of highlighter and shader as separate products in everyday make-up. They are still used in character make-up, particularly in theatrical make-up, where the strong contrast of shades creates the effect.

Applying cream blusher

Cream blusher is usually used in theatrical make-up as the overall effect has to be much stronger because of distance. It is applied with the fingers which does not give the control needed for everyday make-up. The only time cream blusher is used for everyday make-up is in conjunction with powder blusher. For example, if a person loses colour quickly, powder blusher alone is not enough. In such cases, a small amount of cream colour can be blended along the cheek bone immediately after the foundation. Once the powder has then been applied, a second application of powder blusher can be applied over the same area. This will give the colour a much longer staying power.

Applying liquid blusher

Blushers are also available in liquid form. These are best used directly on the skin. Obviously, the skin would then have to be flawless if no foundation was used. The best candidates for this have a tanned skin and therefore do not require foundation. Liquid blusher is applied with the fingers, dotting a little of the colour along the bone and blending it carefully before it dries.

Lipstick

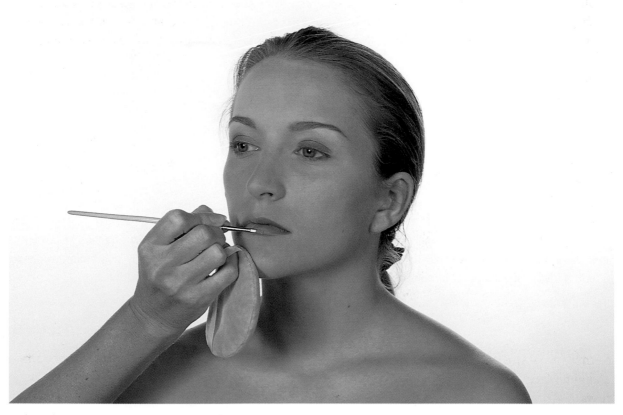

Applying lipstick. Note the correct position of the lip brush

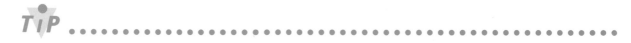

TIP

When first learning to apply lipstick, the best shaped brush is the flat top.

Different textures of lip colour require different sizes of lip brush to apply them correctly. The smaller sized brush is used to apply firmer textures. If the larger brush is used, the shape will distort because of the pressure needed for the harder wax.

Lipstick should be applied in sections, always working towards the centre of the mouth. First, the brush is well loaded with product and flattened. It is then lined up with the lip line and drawn carefully across the edge of the mouth to the centre.

REMEMBER

Too much pressure on the lip brush will distort the shape of the mouth, so be careful that the pressure is firm but not hard.

Lip colour is applied in ten sections (see diagram below) – the corners with the lips slightly apart and the middle sections with the lips together. The only time that the middle sections are applied with the lips apart is when the lips are extremely thin and therefore not fully visible with the lips together. Lipstick is best applied with the lips together because when the lips are apart the muscles relax and the shape therefore alters as the lip brush is moved across them.

Lipstick is applied in ten sections

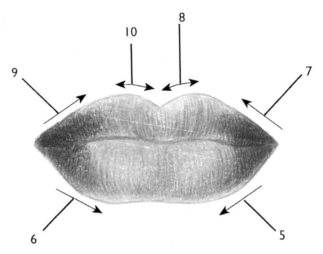

Sections 1–4: Lips apart   Position the flat side of the brush inside the corner of the mouth and align its edge with the edge of the lip line. When the brush touches the lip line, come out towards the centre of the lips by 13 mm (half an inch) and then stop. Continue to fill in the four corners in the same way.

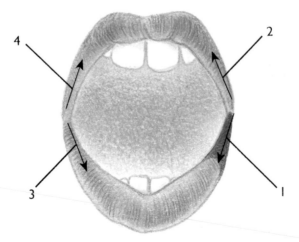

Sections 5–10: Lips together   With the brush in the same position, work towards the centre of the mouth. When the lips are together the muscles around the mouth are not relaxed, therefore the shape will not distort from the pressure of the brush. Too much pressure will distort the shape – the lighter the touch, the better the result.

TIP •

The perfect lip edge will only be achieved if the lip colour is applied with a brush — lip pencils will not create the same precision.

• •

The softer textures of lipstick work better if the lips are dry, although the very soft ones have very little staying power. It is down to the individual make-up artist to decide on the appropriate texture to use, once all the factors have been taken into consideration. Take bridal make-up as an example: the lipstick should have a soft and delicate texture, yet have at least eight hours staying power. How can this be worked out? The answer to this puzzle is easy if you take it one step at a time. Once the colour has been chosen, two textures will need to be used. First, a firmer, matt texture is applied for its staying power. On its own this would be too flat for a young bride who requires a soft, dewy finish. A second layer is therefore applied using a softer texture. This will disappear as everyone kisses the bride, but the matt lipstick will remain visible, which is better than nothing at all.

TIP •

If a second layer of lip colour is applied, particularly of a softer texture, do not take it to the very edge of the first colour — finish it slightly inside, otherwise it may bleed.

• •

Some cosmetic companies have produced a duo lipstick and powder together. The softer texture is dried by applying the powder over it, giving the lipstick a longer staying power. This effect can be achieved with any lipstick by carefully applying a little shadow of the same colour over the surface. If this is tried, do not put the sticky lip brush into the eyeshadow colour or it will damage the shadow. Scrape a little of the shadow off the palate and mix it on the back of the hand with a little lip colour. Loose eyeshadow powder would be easier to use, but the colour range is not as extensive. A slightly frosted shadow gives a better effect.

Lip pencil

There is a common misconception that lip pencils are used to stop lipstick bleeding. This is not the case. In fact, if a lipstick is going to bleed or run, it will do so through any pencil which surrounds it.

Many people, particularly if they have black skin, have what is called a double lip line. This is the area around the lips which is slightly raised. Models often achieve this ridge cosmetically with silicone or collagen which is injected under the skin. If the lips are thin this ridge will not appear, but the illusion can be created by using a lip pencil. The contrast of the darker lip pencil against the paler colour of the skin cleverly duplicates the same effect. The colour of the lip pencil should always be the same or slightly darker than the lipstick colour.

Eye pencil

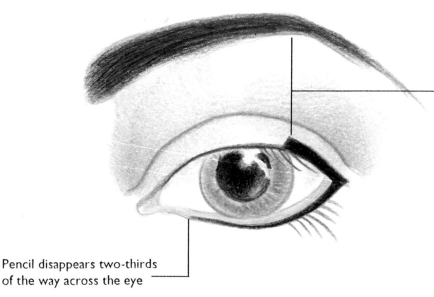

Pencil on the top lid is slightly thicker. It finishes one-third of the way across the eye. When the eye is closed, it comes half way up to the socket line

Pencil disappears two-thirds of the way across the eye

Guidelines for applying eye pencil

TIP ....

Eye pencil should always be set with shadow to stop it creasing.

....

The only area in which eye pencil should be applied is close to the eyelashes. Choosing the correct texture is clearly important because of the delicate tissue around the eyes. The pencil should always be applied using left to right movements in the direction of the nose. The middle finger can be placed at the outer corner of the eye so that the skin does not move with the pencil. Eye pencil must be applied as quickly as possible, or it can make the eyes water. If possible, apply the bottom lid first as it will create a guideline for the top lid when the eye is closed. The eye pencil should be slightly thicker at the outer corner of the eye and disappear the closer it is to the nose.

TIP ....

The best way to blend a pencil is by using a cotton bud.

....

Eyeliner

The most popular colour of eyeliner is black. Eyeliner creates a totally different effect to that of pencil, and is normally applied only to the top lid. The shape drawn can be altered to suit any eye and, on most people, will certainly make the eye appear larger.

Different eyeliner shapes

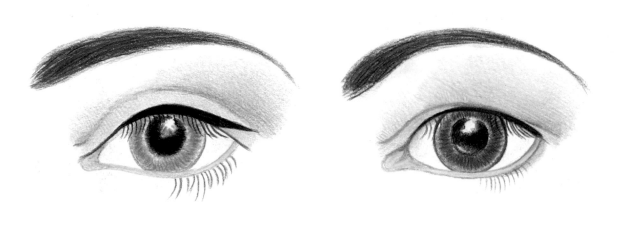

(a) *Eyeliner on an eye with a socket line*   (b) *Eyeliner on an eye without a socket line*

STEP *by* STEP

1 Once the liner brush is loaded with colour, it should be placed on the eyelid at a right angle. In other words, do not point the brush towards the face, but make sure that the full length of the hair has contact with the skin.

2 The brush will then slide along the eyelid to the outer corner. Do not complete the outer corner at this point. That needs to be checked with the eye open to establish the position of the crease line.

3 Once the middle section has been completed and has been left to dry, the eye can be opened and positioned to finish off the corners.

4 With the eye open, the client or model should be asked to look down to the floor – first to the extreme left then to the right.

5 This position will allow the inner corner of the eye to be finished off with a very fine line.

6 The above diagrams show the different shapes that the outer edge can be finished with, particularly if a thick line has been drawn in the middle section.

*M*ascara

Although many models apply their own mascara, salon clients would not be expected to.

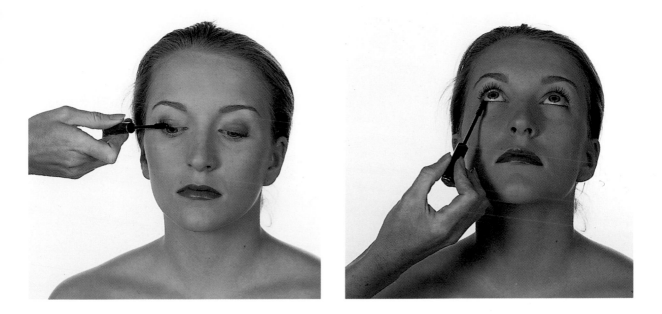

STEP *by* STEP

1. The usual way to apply mascara is by lifting the skin of the eyelid with the client looking down towards the floor.
2. The mascara wand is taken underneath the top lashes and combed through the eyelashes until the amount of product required is built up. (If a client has very sensitive eyes, this particular method is not advisable. The best way to apply the mascara in this instance is to build up the product on top of the lashes first, with the client looking down. The client then cannot see the mascara wand and the eyes are less likely to water.)
3. To apply mascara to the bottom lashes, first remove any excess product from the end of the wand, then use the point to stroke each individual lash. The client should tilt the head slightly and look up to the ceiling, but check that the top lashes do not touch the skin on the top lid.

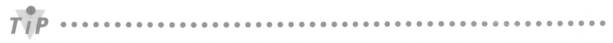

TIP

If a mistake is made, take a cotton bud and point it directly onto the smudge before it has a chance to dry. The motion of rotating it will lift off any mascara. If the mascara has dried, dampen the cotton bud.

False lashes

There are two styles of false lashes; strip and singles. They each give a totally different effect when applied.

Strip lashes

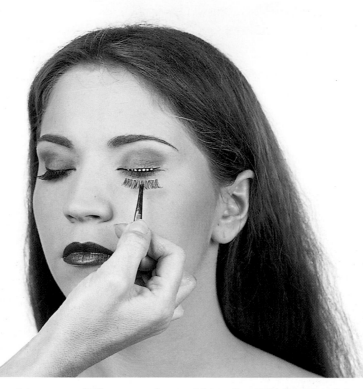

Strip lashes can be found in many different styles and lengths. The width of the strip generally needs to be trimmed to fit the width of the eyelid.

STEP *by* STEP

1. Before the glue is applied to the strip lash, it should be placed along the eyelid and checked for size. The false lashes should start approximately 7 mm (one quarter of an inch) from the corner of the eye, just after the start of the natural lashes. If taken right into the corner of the eye, the strip will feel very uncomfortable for the person wearing it. False lashes take a little getting used to, but after about one hour the client or model will not be aware of them.

2. Trim the eyelashes from the outer edge, which is always the longest.

3. When gluing strip lashes onto the top lid, apply a little of the glue along the eyelid as well as on the lash itself. If the glue is only applied onto the false lash, it will take twice as long to stick – in that time the lash could lift off again if there is a lot of movement from the lid. Take a small amount of glue on the back end of the tweezers and dot it along the top eyelid, as close as possible to the eyelashes without touching the hair.

4 Repeat this on the other eye. This time the gap will allow the glue to become slightly tacky. Once the glue has been applied to the lash itself, it will then hold as soon as it touches the skin.

5 Place the false lashes on the centre of the eyelid and release the tweezers. Make sure that there is no glue on the tweezers before going back to tuck in the corners.

6 The eyelid has a little ridge which curves under before the eyelash hair begins to appear. The strip should be tucked under this ridge at both ends for it to appear perfectly natural.

7 The bottom strip lashes have to be applied under the natural ones. For this reason glue cannot be applied onto the skin, only on the false lash itself.

To remove strip lashes, look down and pull the outer corner of the lash gently – they will just peel off. Remove the old glue and the lashes can be used over and over again. There is no special remover for strip glue. Hold the lash firmly between the fingers and the glue can be carefully picked off.

Single lashes

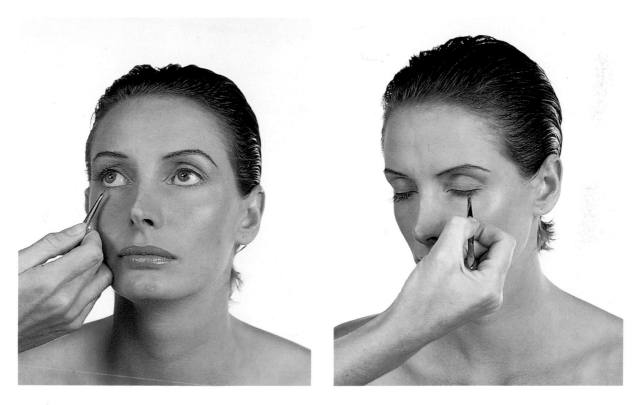

Applying single lashes. Note how the tweezers are held

Single lashes were very popular in the seventies as part of the service that a beauty salon offered. They are available in short, medium, long and under.

REMEMBER

The glue for single lashes should never be substituted for strip lash glue. Single lash glue can only be removed by using a strong chemical remover, which dissolves it. The two different types of glue must therefore *only* be used with the correct lashes, as strip lashes stick to the skin, whereas single lashes are attached to the natural lash itself.

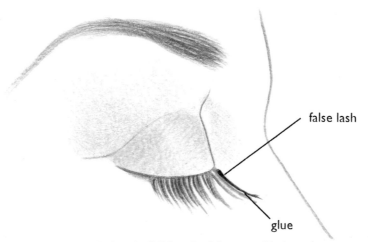

The single false lash should be securely attached to the full length of the natural lash

If the single lashes are applied correctly they should stay attached to the natural eyelashes for approximately six weeks. They are not re-usable.

STEP *by* STEP

1. Most eyelash companies advise that, during single lash application, the client should have the eyes open, looking down. However, in my experience, the single lash glue gives off quite strong fumes which can cause the client's eyes to water. I therefore recommend instead that the client keeps the eyes closed throughout the application. You must, however, get the client to open the eyes for a couple of seconds after every three or four lashes are applied to check that the bottom lashes are completely separate from the top lashes. The glue must not be allowed to dry before the lashes have been checked, and separated if necessary.

2. Dip the end of the single lash into the glue, holding it half way down the shaft with a pair of tweezers. The thumb should always be directly on top of the tweezers for your hand to be in the correct position to apply the false lash. This also applies to strip lashes.

3. Once a bulb of glue has been loaded onto the end of the false lash, it is stroked down the hair of the natural eyelash.

4. The false lash is then positioned on top of the natural lash, as close as possible to the skin but not quite touching. If the false lash touches the skin, it may cause ingrown eyelashes.

5. Once the false lash has been positioned on the natural lash, gently press the lashes together to make sure that the false lash is securely attached to the full length of the real lash.

REMEMBER

It should not be necessary to mascara strip or single lashes. If false lashes have mascara applied to them they will be difficult to clean.

TIP

Always use a non-oily eye make-up remover when wearing single lashes, as any other may dissolve the glue.

Single lashes should stay on for approximately four to six weeks. When the lashes are ready to be removed, take a damp disc of cotton wool and place it underneath the bottom lashes. With the eye closed, dip a cotton bud into the special remover and run it down the lash. This will need to be repeated several times until the glue is dissolved – only then will the lash come away.

Make-up lessons for the client

Clients may also wish to be guided on applying their own make-up. All beauty salons offer make-up lessons as well as make-up application. Once the therapist has worked out which are the best methods and products to use for a particular client, they should be transferred onto a blank face and given to the client for home practice. The client should be given explanations throughout the make-up lesson as to why certain products have been used and also why particular techniques will work best for her. If the therapist fully understands all of the areas covered in this book, there will be no difficulty in answering any questions which may arise.

SUMMARY POINTS (ADJUSTING YOUR MISTAKES)

- If the blusher colour is too heavy, especially near the eye, remove it with a clean, dry wedge.
- If the blusher has emphasized any skin problems, remove it as above. Then rebuild the colour using alternate layers of powder and blusher.
- If mascara smudges – *stop immediately* – and remove it with a clean cotton bud. Never allow mascara to dry on the skin.
- Never use single lash glue for strip lashes, and vice versa.

Questions

1 When would you use an eyebrow pencil instead of an eyebrow shadow?

2 If mascara smudges onto the skin, how is it best removed?

3 How can eyeshadow be made to appear more vibrant?

4 How can you cover dark circles around the eyes?

5 How would you cover a scar or birthmark?

6 How do you prevent eyeshadow from creasing?

5

Colour and light

KEY AREAS

At the end of this chapter you will know about:

- Choosing colour to achieve the desired outcome with the client
- The effect of light and dark on faces

Colour

Most people are totally confused when it comes to choosing the right colours – whether wearing them or applying them. I have always found it much easier to give basic guidelines and leave the experimenting to those who have an eye for colour. For simplicity, colour can be divided into two categories: warm and cold (sometimes described as natural and synthetic).

Using colour

These colour groupings can be used in two ways. Generally one group is chosen and then used consistently for the eyes, lips and cheeks. This, in fact, is the safest way to work. However, if you look at the daring of the fashion designers, you will see that they use the opposite groups together and create fabulous collections. I have personally experimented with colour over the past few years, although when I first came into the make-up business I stuck rigidly to one group or the other. After using both in different ways, I have found that I prefer the effect of contrasting colour.

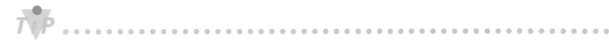

The lips and cheeks must have the same tones for contrasting colour to work successfully.

If, for example, someone is wearing shades of grey and pink, using greys and pinks in their make-up can look very flat. Stick to the greys on the eyes, but use peaches for the lips and cheeks – you will find that the whole face lights up. The difference can be amazing. Always try and keep the eyes neutral, as using a contrasting colour in that area, which is bright, would be a disaster on a normal make-up. Quite often cosmetic companies produce advertisements where all the colours of the rainbow seem to be mixed together. This may look fabulous, but remember that the model they are using is likely to be young and have flawless skin.

Warm (natural) colours　　　　　　*Cold (synthetic) colours*

Examples of colours from the two tone spectrums are shown above. Most of the colours are duplicated – it is their undertones which vary. Unfortunately there are no hard and fast rules on which colour groups to use. I can give you guidelines and questions to ask yourself before deciding, but in the end the choice comes down to trial and error, and your own judgement as to what looks right.

Matching colour

Students frequently ask me if the eye colour is important, but today this has little relevance in deciding what colours to use. The main areas which should influence your choice of colour are the clothes, the hair and the skin tone.

Fashion designers have mixed warm reds and cool pinks with much success. If this sort of combination is worn do not even consider trying to match the colour of the clothes, look at the hair or skin tone instead. The importance of the hair and skin will also become apparent if the client is wearing a plain black evening gown, or for a bride in all white.

Generally the hair will only influence the choice if the colour is dominant, for example red. The skin tone will either have warm or cold undertones. If the skin tone has cool undertones, then it may need the warmth of natural colour. Conversely, if the skin has warm undertones, it may appear too orange if natural colour is applied.

If the eye make-up is neutral (this can be achieved with all of the dark shades by applying a black pencil underneath them), then the only colour to decide upon will be the lips and cheeks.

REMEMBER

Don't be frightened to experiment with colour slowly and carefully over a period of time. There are always groupings that you can fall back on, particularly if you follow my guidelines.

Client make-up is the most difficult when deciding upon the right colour match. Working on models is completely different – they are specifically chosen so that their colouring and looks are right for the style which is to be created.

The classic look

There is a make-up which can be classed as colourless; the classic red lips, black liner and false lashes. We have seen this colourless classic in many different situations – Marilyn Monroe depicted the look perfectly, as did Madonna.

STEP *by* STEP

1. The base for this classic look needs to be flawless – cream foundation gives the best effect.
2. The eyebrows have to be perfectly shaped as they are taking the place of the shadow.
3. The thickness of the liner will depend on the position of the socket line. If the socket line is deep then the eyeliner can be applied slightly more thickly. If the socket line is barely visible then the liner would be much thinner.
4. False eyelashes finish off the eyes.
5. The lip colour should be true red.

No blusher is used in this look as it is not appropriate and will detract from the dramatic effect. This make-up is obviously a model look, but young clients with good features will do it justice. It is simple, but very effective.

Black skin

Chapter 7 deals with black skin in more detail, but as a general rule follow exactly the same guidelines as for any colour skin. Group the colours into warm and cold, not forgetting the neutral or colourless look which is fabulous on a black skin.

REMEMBER

Don't treat black skin differently: stop, think, and take it section by section – breaking down each step as with any other make-up.

TIP

When I first worked on black skin, I pretended that I was working on someone with a very good tan.

All the colour tests are the same as for white skin; the hair is predominantly black, the skin tones have very obvious undertones, cold or warm, and the clothes must be taken into consideration. The main difference to the total make-up (and this also applies to someone with a dark tan) is that the complexion should not be completely matt, otherwise it will look grey. This is easily dealt with by adding coloured or frosted powders at the end of the make-up (see chapter 2).

Certain people do have an eye for colour. I can choose colours and know that they are right, but it is very difficult to explain the choice. If you find you do not have this gift, just stick to the guidelines and you will not go far wrong.

Light

Effects of light and dark

When I talk about light, I do not mean lighting techniques. The ordinary make-up artist should not need to understand any of the technical details of lighting – leave this to the lighting experts.

What I do want to talk about is how light and dark colours affect the overall look of the make-up. The basic guideline is that light emphasizes and dark takes away or detracts. This is true in most areas when applying make-up. However, the reverse can create a much better effect.

Light and dark (or highlighting and shading) has always been the term used when sculpting the face. Most make-up books illustrate various different face shapes, for example square, triangular, round, etc., where any area outside the perfect oval should be shaded away. Today this technique is only used for theatrical or character make-up. It is not used in straight television or photographic and fashion make-up, and most certainly not in everyday make-up.

Special effects: what can't be achieved

Do not be taken in by magazine articles which state that a double chin will disappear if shaded brown, or that a wide nose will appear slimmer if shaded down either side. Think about it – the shaded feature will simply look dirty and more obvious than if you had done nothing to it at all. We do not stand fifty yards away from a person to hold a conversation, so the true features will always show through the make-up.

REMEMBER

Make-up can emphasize the good points and detract from the bad, it can even create illusion, but it cannot make things disappear.

Special effects: what can be achieved

Light and dark colours can make features more prominent and thereby make others appear relatively less obvious.

Foundation

Mature skin will look younger if it is slightly darker. An older client will age about ten years if a pale foundation is applied. It is better to take a shade which is slightly darker than the natural skin colour. Do not worry about the jawline – this can be blended away using a slightly lighter foundation at the edge, or a wedge which is slightly dampened with moisturizer. The only other alternative is to darken the foundation by applying a darker tinted powder at the end of the make-up. This would avoid the problems of using a darker foundation.

Blusher

Blushers come in light and dark shades and you must be careful where each is applied. Darker ones are always applied underneath the cheek bone – if applied too high they will give the illusion that the area which should be prominent is sinking in.

If you are using blusher for shape then two colours should be used, the heavier one at the baseline. Paler blushers on their own are used to add colour, but that is all. In this case the face would need good cheek bones to create its own shape.

Lipstick

Lipstick can be problematic. Take, for example, thin lips; they need a pale colour to make them appear larger but, if the colour is too pale, the lips will not be seen at all. This is when a lip pencil is useful. Outlining the lips with a slightly darker shade will make them appear slightly larger and they can then be filled in with the paler colour. Use a lip brush to bleed the edges of the pencil and the lipstick together.

Black women have rather full lips which, in theory, should make you choose a dark colour lipstick. However, if the lipstick chosen is too dark, the colour will not be visible. Many black women use a slightly paler lip colour which looks beautiful, especially if it is frosted.

Eye colour

The guideline (light emphasizes and dark takes away) does not work for the eyes. In fact, the darker the eye make-up, the more prominent the eyes become. This can be seen immediately with the use of eyeliner.

The problem when using dark eye colours is that most people deal with them in the same way they do paler colours, and unfortunately this does not work. Dark eyeshadow has to be very precise. One side of the colour should be blended well, but the other side should be kept in a solid line – otherwise the effect created is of a black eye.

There will be more information in this book on tones of colour, light, medium and dark. I hope, however, that this brief chapter has made some of the myths about light and dark clearer.

SUMMARY POINTS

- When choosing which colours to use, check what colour the client is wearing, then their skin tone, then their hair colour.
- Lips and cheeks should be colour co-ordinated with the same tones.
- Remember that make-up has limitations – you can only make the best of what you have to start with.

Questions

1 How can you make the eyes appear larger?

2 What are the easiest categories to divide colour into?

3 On what areas of the face should the colours always be co-ordinated?

4 When applying the eyeshadow on an older woman, what guidelines should be followed when choosing colour?

6
Make-up styles

Now that the technical details about the textures of cosmetic products and their methods of application have been covered, I would like to put the information into practise. Once the techniques have been put together, different make-up styles can be created. These methods can be used in any aspect of straight make-up. Unfortunately, you cannot follow a set pattern for every look, because each person has their own style, features, skin tones and hair colour. I will recommend step-by-step guidelines, but the final decision will always be up to you.

REMEMBER

Anyone can learn to apply make-up. Styles have to be created.

The Linda Meredith STEP *by* STEP guide

1. Check the skin with the back of the hand. It should have the same feeling as the skin on the inside of the forearm.
2. Check the colour match of the foundation. (Apply three shades of foundation across the forehead or any other clear area on the face. Any colour change will occur within the first few minutes.)
3. Apply moisturizer on the face and halfway down the neck.
4. Apply the foundation while the moisturizer is still tacky. (If the foundation has a high oil content, let the moisturizer absorb into the skin first.)
5. Stipple on the powder, working on one section until it is completely dry before moving to the next

6 Shape the eyebrow hair with a comb, pencil or shadow if required. (The eyebrows should have been plucked before the make-up is started.)

7 Apply a pale base colour over the entire eyelid.

8 Draw a black pencil line three-quarters of the way under the bottom lid and one-quarter of the way over the top lid. The colour on the top lid should be slightly thicker. Blend with a cotton bud.

9 Set the pencil line with a dark shadow. On the top lid only, take the shadow up to the crease line.

10 With a medium shadow, lightly blend across the eyelid above the crease line. (This must be carried out with the eye open.)

11 Close the eye and blend the two colours into one another.

12 Apply the lip colour which has been chosen.

13 Return to the eyes and apply liner and mascara (or liner and false eyelashes if used).

14 Apply blusher to match the lip colour.

This is my basic step-by-step guide which can be used on any face. Varying the shades of colour and their depth will alter this look to suit every occasion. The guidelines will be referred to throughout the rest of this chapter.

Background note

It is interesting to look back over the fashions in colour cosmetics, to understand better the look we have arrived at in the nineties. The eighties gave us a society which was very health conscious. Clothes had softer lines and were easy to wear. This healthy, relaxed way of living was complemented with a soft, natural make-up. Foundation became sheer, revealing a healthy glow; mascara lost its fibres to give a softer, more natural appearance. Lips lost their colour but seemed to increase in size with the use of lip pencils, while eyebrows had never seen such freedom.

The seventies were dominated by a strong dramatic fashion look, where anything that was tight or shiny was vogue. Every different type of cosmetic was heavily laden with frost or glitter. The aim was to apply as many different eyeshadow colours as possible. Glitter would link the eyes and the cheeks together and, although lip colours were strong, the lips appeared thinner.

Sixties fashion was heavily dominated by black and white and, in some ways, this effect seemed to be reflected in the face. Eyes would be ringed in black (in those days they used carbon black, in other words soot) or show bold unblended lines. They would also be surrounded on either side with several layers of false eyelashes. This dramatic effect was maintained by the lack of lipstick and blusher. When blusher was applied it was flanked either side by highlighter and shader. Looking back, the overall effect was rather mask-like due to the base which was a heavy, pale wax.

Max Factor and Ponds dominated the fifties. The looks they created were simple, but effective. Foundation and powder had not yet attained individual identities. Nevertheless, together they produced a dry but effective base. Eyes were finely lined with black, but rarely saw more than one colour. The priority on the face was undoubtedly the lips. Lipstick was matt and heavily laden with pigment which gave tremendous staying power. The problems which arose with later lipsticks were unheard of then. The periods béfore this revolution of the cosmetic industry had their individual style, but never with the influence that followed.

Cosmetic camouflage

Cosmetic camouflage is the term used when severe skin disorders need to be concealed before the application of any style of make-up. It can be split into two very different areas. The first and most technical is usually carried out within a hospital. For example, a prosthesis may be required if part of the face has been severely destroyed, usually by cancer. Special materials are moulded and coloured to match the shape and tone of the area that is no longer there. A false eye or a dental plate may need to be fitted within the prosthesis. If a particular hospital specializes in this type of work, a cosmetic camouflage technician would probably be part of the hospital staff – otherwise the Red Cross have people who work in this field.

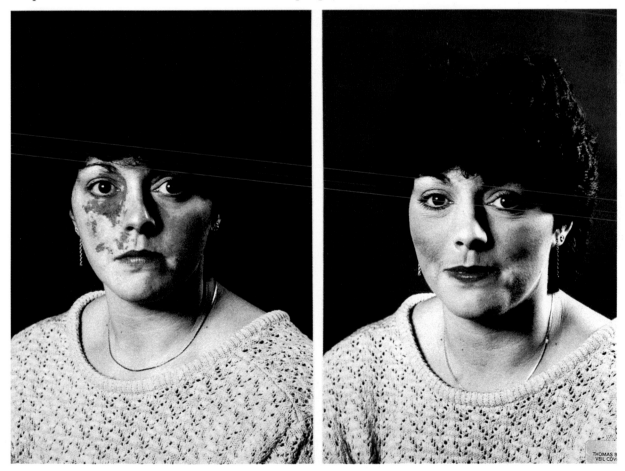

Using cosmetic camouflage to cover a port-wine stain

The second area of cosmetic camouflage deals with skin disorders such as port-wine stains or vitiligo. This type of problem can be easily dealt with by the therapist. The most popular product for cosmetic camouflage is called Veil. The application of this product is basically the same as for any other foundation, and any of the foundation application methods can be used. There are, however, some important differences. The first is that no moisturizer should be applied to the skin first, otherwise the product will not adhere to the skin properly. Secondly, the product is waterproof and will not wear off the skin like any normal foundation. It can only be removed with a cleanser.

The product comes in various shades which can be used individually or mixed to match the skin tone exactly. The product should be applied thinly as it has been formulated to give complete coverage. It can be blended over the entire face instead of using another foundation with it. However, if you decide to use an ordinary foundation over the rest of the face, make sure that it contains a high water content. Too much oil in the product may weaken the covering power of the camouflage product.

For extra staying power, Veil has a waterproof powder which can be used to set the foundation. Once applied, the usual colour products can be blended in the same way over the surface to create the finished look.

Day and evening make-up

I have purposely linked these two looks together. Most people have a particular style which they like, and few will change to something completely different when it comes to the evening.

Young skin

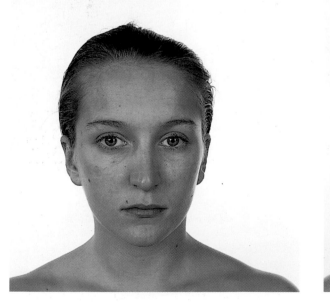
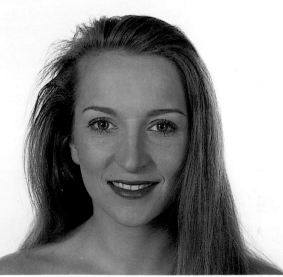

Day make-up

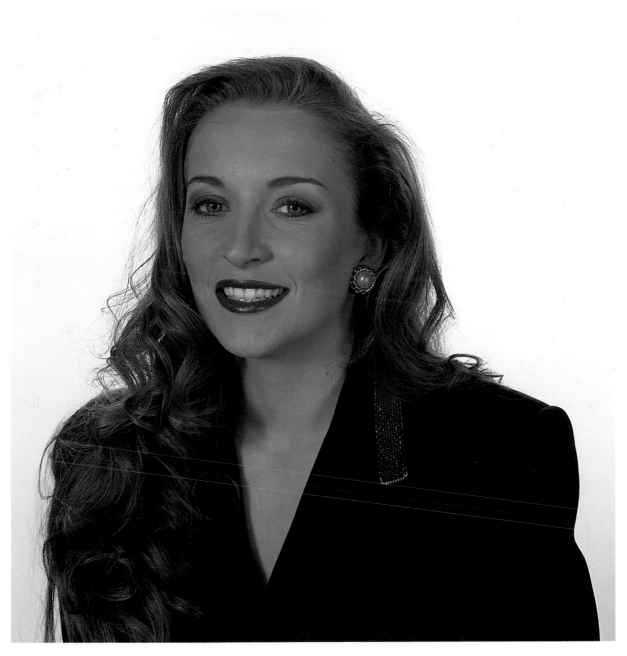

Evening make-up

STEPS TO NOTE

- All 14 steps are important.

These photographs show a glamorous make-up that can be used for both day and evening. The style is a classic look which will suit most women and can be altered in depth to create a softer or stronger look. A change in outfit and hair style will complete the final look.

Middle-aged skin

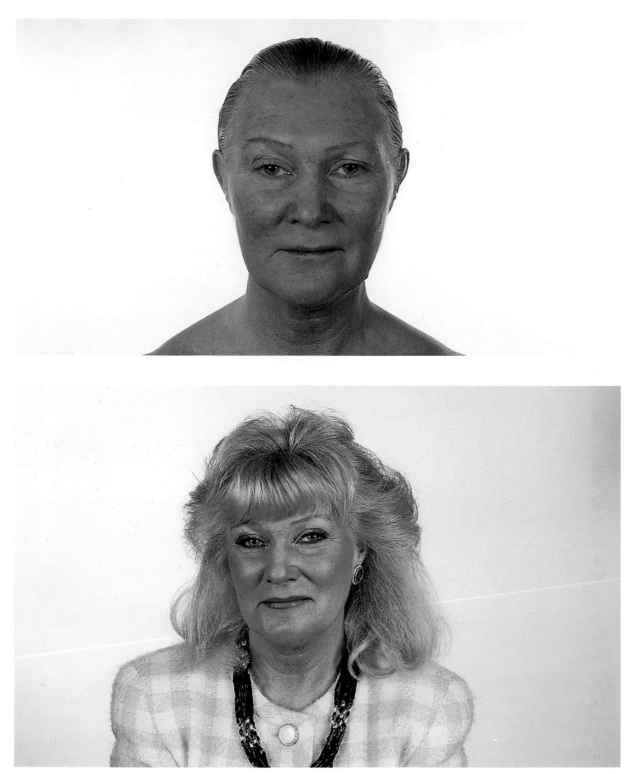

Day make-up

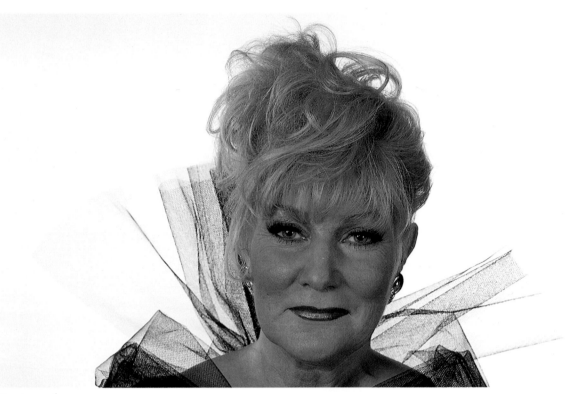

Evening make-up

STEPS TO NOTE

- **Step 2** – Pay particular attention to this step. The foundation may look better one shade darker, especially if the client has a florid complexion.
- **Step 4** – The foundation should be applied as thinly as possible.
- **Step 5** – Do not overload the eye area with powder, but make sure it is completely dry or the eyeshadow will smudge.
- **Step 6** – Shadow can be used on the existing hair but, to match the depth of colour, draw the tail end with an eyebrow pencil.
- **Step 7** – The pale eye-base should not be too frosted.
- **Step 12** – If the lipstick has a tendency to bleed, use a harder wax and apply the soft texture over the top, but do not take it right to the edge.
- **Step 14** – Check the blusher guidelines. If the face is too thin, bring the colour in towards the iris of the eye.

The method of application remains the same for the client who is over forty. The main variation for this age group is the thickness of the foundation. A heavier base will accentuate lines and therefore age the person. The foundation should be applied more thinly and a shade darker than the natural skin tone. If this is difficult, because of the colouring of the skin on the neck and body, then the colour can be changed by applying a darker powder at the end of the make-up. The evening look is exaggerated with false eyelashes which make the eyes appear larger.

Mature skin

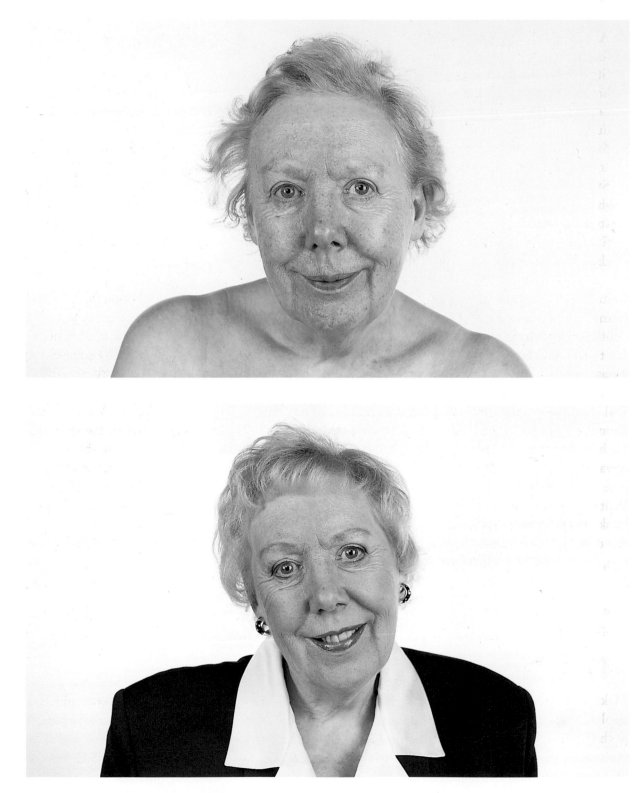

STEPS TO NOTE

- All steps to take particular care with are the same as for middle-aged skin, except the following:
- **Step 2** – Take particular care when matching foundation. Again a shade darker will look healthier, but watch the skin colour on the neck and chest – it may be what is called 'turkey neck', which means it will be very red and mottled. This must be taken into consideration during the colour choice.
- **Step 5** – If a very thin layer of foundation has been applied, compact powder will be adequate to set it so as not to emphasize too many lines.
- **Steps 9 and 10** – Make sure that the skin is stretched to its maximum when applying the shadow in step 9. When applying step 10 let the skin relax to apply the last colour, but then stretch it to blend the two colours together.
- **Step 13** – Lift the skin on the eyelid straight up (not out to the side) until the lashes lift slightly. The skin will then be smooth enough to draw in the eyeliner.

Mature women should be separated into two categories – the glamorous older woman and the homely, more conventional type. Colour products chosen for both women should be more subtle, for example shades of grey, browns, burgundy and, of course, black, which is fabulous for the glamorous looks. Bright vibrant colours should definitely not be used as the look they create would be more along the lines of fantasy. The darker the shadow, the more effective the results in diminishing crêpey eyelids. This, however, would make the more conventional woman feel over-made-up. In this situation the client must be consulted as to how strongly the shadows should be applied, so that she is comfortable with the effect. No matter how strong the shadow, both looks are best finished off with the correct thickness of liquid eyeliner. Blushers should always be shown as part of the face, not something that has just been added at the last minute. The colour should be of a soft shade chosen from the natural or warm groups, and should be kept away from the centre of the face which may be highly coloured due to the presence of tiny broken capillaries. Lipstick colours should be chosen from the same family as the blusher, but the depth may need to balance with the depth of the eye shadow. As lips can appear thinner with age, the lips will appear fuller if they are lined with a lip pencil.

The main factor shown in all of these make-ups is balance. This means that the depth of colour overall is applied to complement each feature.

REMEMBER

Make sure one particular feature does not overpower the others. This is very important when applying straight make-up – so often the blusher seems to dominate the whole face. Always look at the finished make-up as a whole.

Wedding make-up

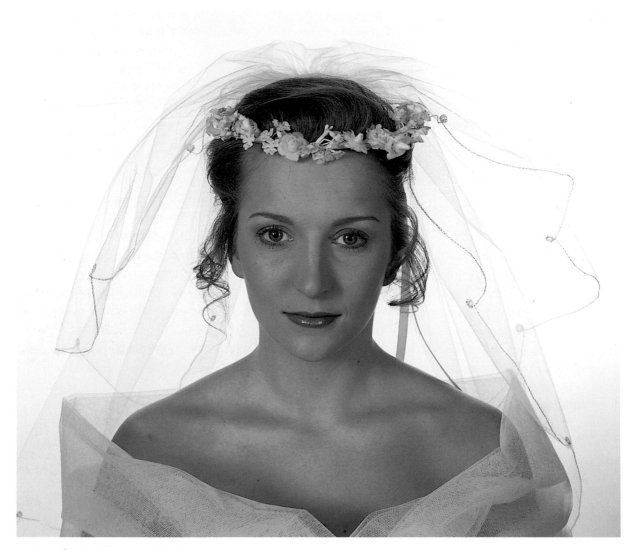

Make-up for the classic young bride

STEPS TO NOTE

- All 14 steps are followed but particular attention is paid to **Step 12** as the lipstick should stay all day. Apply the hard wax texture first and then the glossy one over the top.
- **Step 13** – Single eyelashes are perfect for a wedding make-up as they will stay on right through the honeymoon (if applied correctly).

The above photograph shows the classic young bride (although we all know that bridal make-up can easily apply to someone much older, who may be tying the knot for the third or fourth time). The step-by-step guide to the basic format can be adapted very successfully here, but I have chosen to show you a variation which is well suited to this look.

Preparation and base

The texture of the foundation will depend on the coverage needed. The initial steps for the preparation and the base through to the eyebrows is the same as for the other styles. The base on the eyelid should be a pale colour, with either a hint of pink or a hint of peach in it.

Colour combinations

The colours of the bridesmaids' dresses and the flowers can be taken into consideration when choosing colour combinations for the bride. If the colouring is peach or yellow, then warm shades can be used. If, however, they are pink or blue, then cool shades can be used. Do not forget to also check the skin tone and hair colouring of the bride herself.

Eye make-up

Once the base colour has been applied, a pencil should be used (black is still suitable) in a very thin line through the top and bottom lashes. This will emphasize them slightly and give the overall eye make-up a much longer staying power.

After blending it well with a cotton bud so that it has the appearance of being grey rather than black, add a soft grey shadow over the pencil to set it, both on the top lid and the bottom lid. A medium contrast, either a slightly deeper peach or a neutral pink (not vibrant) is then applied right across the eyelid above the grey. Check, with the eyes open, that enough of the two shades can be seen – if not add a little more.

Lip make-up

The lips are the biggest problem. Everyone will want to kiss the bride and we do not want the lip colour to disappear totally before the photographs are taken. Although lipstick can always be touched up throughout the reception, it would be advisable to apply the lipstick in such a way that it has a little more staying power. For the type of eye make-up we have chosen, a soft, delicate colour of lipstick would be better suited to blend with the overall look. Unfortunately, these lipsticks are usually made of a soft texture and will therefore disappear quite quickly.

TIP

The best way to add the extra staying power needed is to first apply a hard wax lipstick of a similar pale colour. The soft one may still disappear slightly, but the balance of the overall look will be maintained.

Finishing touches

A very thin line of eyeliner is applied tightly on top of the lashes and, to finish the look completely, three or four single lashes can be added to the outer corners.

A hint of blusher should be applied on top of the cheek bones to add a little colour to the skin. This should always match the lip colour.

Depending on the cut of the dress, a little foundation may be needed over the neck and shoulder area. If you have a 'blushing bride', there is a possibility that the chest may flush with colour. In that case, take a small amount of foundation directly onto the wedge and blend it down the neck, over the shoulders and across the chest. Set it with a little powder, applied with the powder brush.

This look is perfect for the young bride, and one which she will be totally comfortable with.

Photographic make-up

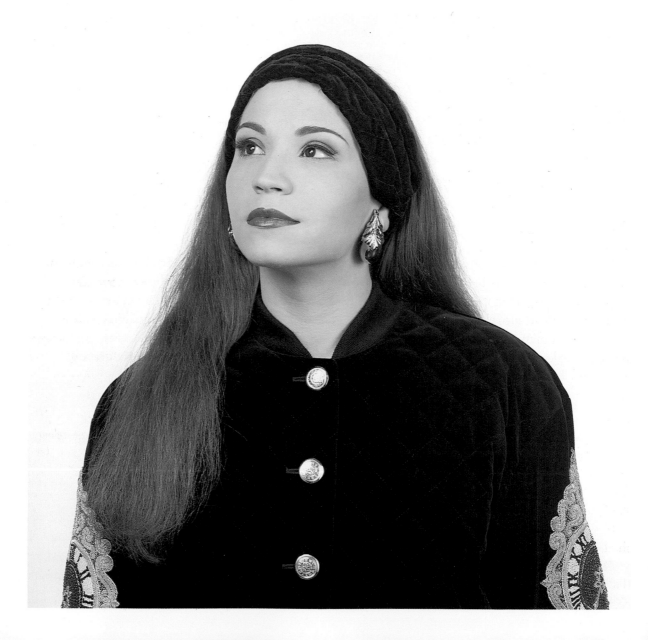

STEPS TO NOTE

- **Step 2** – In photographic make-up, it is not always necessary to have the identical colour match with the foundation. The look may require a colour change if no part of the body is shown. If this is the case, then a colour test is not necessary.
- **Step 3** – If the foundation has movement in it (for example a wax, or one with a high oil content), a moisturizer is not always necessary because the make-up is removed as soon as the photograph is taken.
- **Step 5** – Make sure enough powder is used to allow the make-up to last throughout the session, without having to retouch.
- The first five steps are followed, but the colour section may be altered depending on the final look required. For example, some looks are completely without blusher, or a fashion look may show the blusher only in the centre of the face.

REMEMBER

Whatever is applied, it needs to be as perfect as possible – otherwise the camera will pick up any flaws, especially if the shot is for a close-up beauty look.

Photographic tricks of the trade

Photographic make-up can cover so many styles and variations that several chapters could be dedicated to it alone.

Most magazine photographs that we see today have been re-touched. For example, famous film stars are often used to advertise cosmetic ranges and perfumes – these may show their features at close proximity, yet they appear flawless. Such perfection might be expected of the younger super models, but not of actresses over forty. Age lines, an uneven complexion, or even the odd blemish would certainly be seen in the flesh. This is not a problem for the make-up artist to deal with; instead it is left to the re-toucher. Re-touching is a big business and can command fees of up to £250 an hour. The therapist working on clients in a salon will have to deal with the main repercussions of this industry. Many clients will use these pictures for reference when having make-up applied. In their innocence, they believe such perfection can be achieved with make-up. This of course is not so.

Another procedure that the photographer can use is filtering. A small mesh is placed over the camera lens which creates a slightly blurry image, depending on the thickness of the mesh. (In the days of the famous photographer Parkinson, this same effect was achieved using a nylon stocking.) The blurry image softens age lines.

Good photographers are also experts in lighting techniques which can be used to shape or shade the face with fine precision.

Techniques in photographic make-up have changed enormously over the last few decades. All the make-up artist has to do is create the look which they wish to see in the photograph, the rest is down to the photographer. It is the photographer's job to produce a photograph which is a duplicate of what can be seen on the model's face. Unfortunately, however, there are still many photographers working with dated techniques which can bleach out the make-up that has been applied.

TiP ·······································

When working with photographers for the first time, I always discuss beforehand how heavy they would like me to apply the make-up. If their response is 'just do what you wish to see', then I know that they are up to date and understand what they are doing.

·······································

Modelling styles

Models are chosen for their looks and features. (I remember once choosing a model for the shape of her mouth, everything else was irrelevant.) There is no set style to follow. It could entail making up a model's hands for a nail polish advertisement, or applying body make-up for a deodorant company. This is why the make-up artist is always briefed on what the job entails beforehand.

The application methods for photographic make-up are no different to the methods that we use every day, the difference is in how they are put together to create a look.

Black-and-white photographic make-up

There are commonly misconceptions about how to deal with the make-up for black-and-white photography. Most fashion and beauty photographers shoot black-and-white and colour pictures at the same time. There are, in fact, very few colour prints that would not be acceptable if run off in black and white. An easy way to check is to run a colour photograph through a copy machine – this will give you a good idea of what it would look like in black and white.

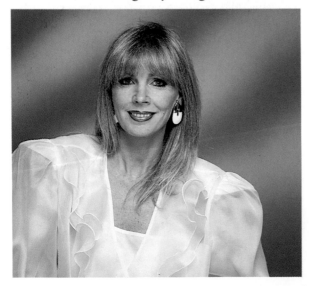
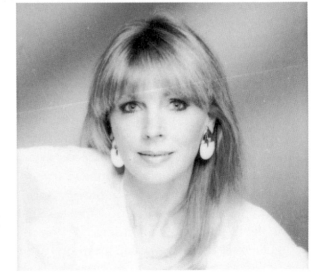

Compare these two photographs – taken within five minutes of each other

STEPS TO NOTE

- The first five steps are to be followed as for colour photographic make-up.
- Once onto the colour section, the main point to remember is contrast when choosing the colours. This is in relation to the skin which is the base.
- Remember, the eyes will only show white, grey and black. The eye steps listed are perfect for black and white shots, because, if followed, they do show contrast.
- **Step 14** – Blusher is the main area to be careful with. If the colour chosen is too dark and is applied on the cheek bone, it will produce the opposite effect from that intended and make the cheek bone appear to sink in instead of standing out. If the colour chosen is much darker than the skin, it should be applied underneath the bone and not over it. Follow the same guidelines but work 25 mm (one inch) up from the baseline instead of 50 mm (two inches).

REMEMBER

All you have to consider is contrast. Think black, grey and white, because that is all that will be shown.

The basic technique, using the shades of light, medium and dark, will work perfectly well for any black-and-white shots. Every colour that is applied should be in contrast to the skin colour. The shape of the face and blusher can be easily defined with the photographer's lighting, although, if a darker blusher is used, it should be applied under the cheek bone. Black and white make-up is as simple as that.

Applying blusher for black-and-white photographic make-up

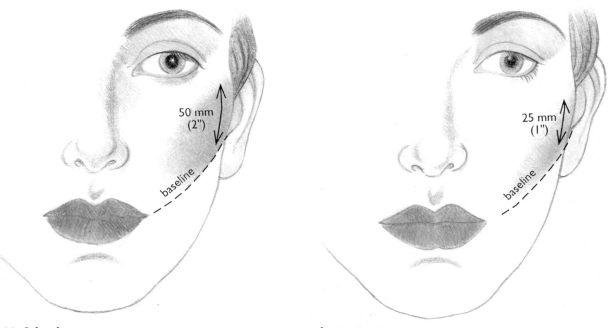

(a) *Pale colour*　　　　　　　　　　　　　　　　(b) *Dark colour*

Fashion make-up

The fashion industry is closely linked to the seasons — with every season a new look is created. The colours and styles of the clothes designed dictate the fashion of make-up. Earlier in this chapter I briefly mentioned the changes in fashion over the last decades and how they influenced the make-up. When creating any kind of make-up, even on a salon client, their style and dress must always be taken into consideration.

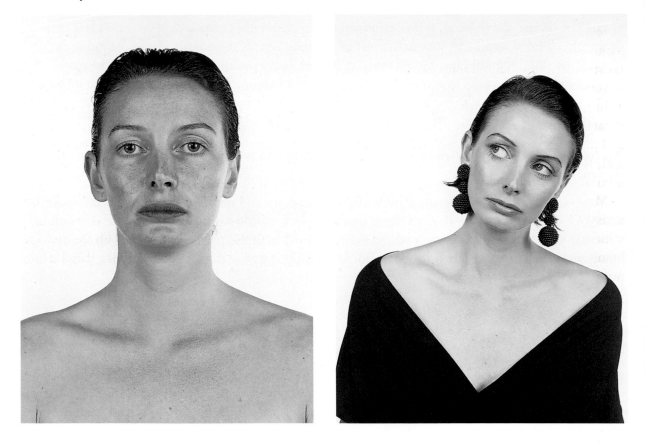

STEPS TO NOTE

- Fashion make-up has always been for the young. When a certain age is reached, the classic more conventional looks should prevail.
- Cosmetic companies will change their colour products each season to complement fashion trends, but stick to the darker muted shades for the older clients.
- Colour co-ordination is generally reversed in fashion make-up. As long as the eyes are kept to neutral shades try using colours on the lips and cheeks which contrast with what the client is wearing. You will be surprised at the result.
- False eyelashes will go in and out of fashion with each season. If the overall effect is better with them, then use them.

REMEMBER

Clients visiting a beauty salon may ask for a fashion make-up without really realizing what the fashion is at that point in time. The classic glamour look is more likely what they have in mind.

Fashion shows

Freelance make-up artists are used for all the top shows. The designers tend to use the same make-up artists over and over again – they are reluctant to change when they have built up a trust in them and their ability. Some of the models apply their own make-up, if the look required is not something out of the ordinary.

In the past, fashion make-up might have been classed as heavy, sometimes bordering on theatrical. This, in fact, depends totally on the show. Most shows nowadays have the audience and press very close to the catwalk. The press may use some of these photos in their releases and, because the camera picks up everything at this level, the make-up must therefore look natural and not too theatrical.

Make-up for fashion shows must be perfect and simple, but effective. The aim of the make-up artist is to bring out the model's features, rather like the mannequins that we see in store windows. It should be sharp and precise, but the priority is always that it works with the clothes being shown. Certain aspects of fashion make-up are designed only to create a look, they are not expected to be followed.

REMEMBER

The fashion designer will create a catwalk show just for the press attention. Most of the looks will never be seen in the shops.

Magazine fashion

Fashion make-up is seen in magazines as well as on the catwalk. This is handled in the same way as photographic make-up, bearing in mind that the camera will pick up every detail. Application methods are the same throughout – they must be applied with care so they remain as perfect as possible until they are removed.

TIP

Bearing in mind the recent revival of the seventies glitter, it is important that the make-up artist has an extensive kit to meet any demand.

Fantasy make-up

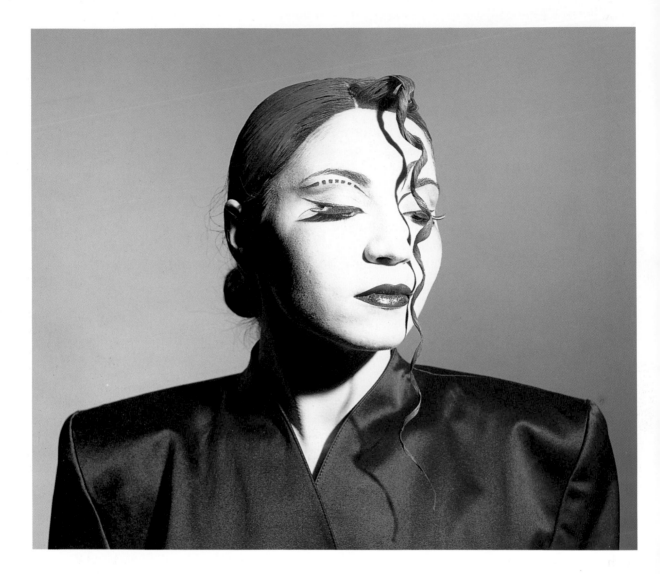

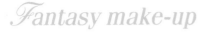 **STEPS TO NOTE**

- Anything goes.
- If the detail is to be drawn onto a base (as in the above example), the first five steps should be followed, but not necessarily the colour match as the effect is better on a pale base.
- Aqua colour is used to draw the detail, but if the face has to be coloured then it is used in place of the foundation.
- As regards detail of colour, any design can be created, but the methods of application for each product should be followed.

Fantasy make-up is the one area of make-up where anything goes. It is used occasionally for television commercials or for advertising particular products. A recent advertising campaign showing fantasy make-up was by Pirelli, the tyre company. It was used for their 1992 calendar, which depicted the twelve animals of the Chinese calendar.

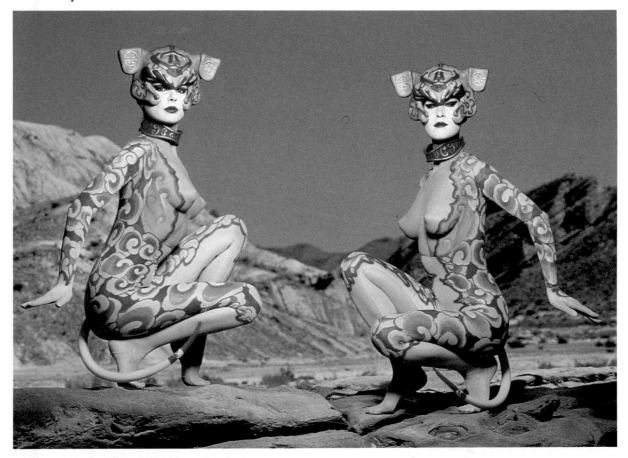

Fantasy make-up used in the 1992 Pirelli calendar

The overall effect was superb – the lower part of the body was covered with specially printed tights, which was then matched by the make-up on the upper part of the body. Elaborate headdresses were used to depict the features of each animal. The calendar took a week on location to shoot, at enormous expense, but the overall effect certainly paid off.

Fantasy make-up is the most artistic area of professional make-up, as the make-up is literally painted onto the face or body. There are make-up artists who specialize in this kind of make-up, and it is without doubt an art form. I have even seen coke cans, burgers and fruit drawn onto the body, creating the most amazing effects. Some of these make-ups can take up to twelve hours to apply – how sad when they can be cleaned off in a matter of minutes.

The products used to create these effects are either water or oil based. The most popular make is Kryolan which has in its range Aqua colour and Super colour, ideal for fantasy make-up. They can be applied with damp sponges, or with a fine eyeliner brush if detail is required. The professional make-up shops carry all of these specialized products.

Character make-up

Character make-up for the theatre

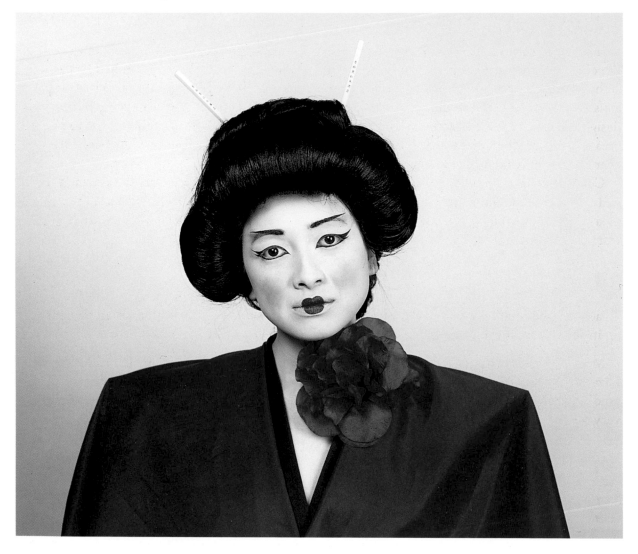

- If character make-up is to be achieved using latex, then the guidelines should obviously not be followed.
- If the character is to be created using wax, then this is applied directly on the skin and no colour test is necessary.
- All wax products should be applied before any powder is put on, to create the desired effect.
- The method of product application is as shown in chapter 4.

TiP

One advantage of character make-up for the theatre is that it does not have to be as perfect as the other styles because of the distance between the stage and the audience.

Character make-up is used to change the appearance of a person, to aid them in the portrayal of the character they are playing. In most theatrical productions the make-up is applied by the actors themselves, a useful skill which they learn as part of their training. Although make-up artists may not be used for the actual application of the make-up, they will certainly be used to design the look of the character. A make-up artist will also be brought in if the effects to be created are not straightforward. For example, in the production of *Phantom of the Opera*, the character requires an effect which can only be achieved by using latex.

Character make-up used in the theatre is generally achieved using wax products, which are still the easiest and quickest to apply if two shows a day are being performed. This is the one area of make-up which has remained heavy. In fact, close up theatrical make-up can look terrible, but you have to remember that it is applied for distance.

REMEMBER

To achieve the total look of any character, the hair and costumes are as important as the make-up itself. In fact, it cannot be successfully achieved without all three.

Most characters are created using the same basic make-up, which is usually the pale base. Elizabeth I, the Mikado, Copelia, and many more all have a similar base. It is only the detail used for the features which changes the overall character. If you can perfect one, the others are very easy to create.

TiP

Many amateur productions take on make-up artists. Don't expect to be paid for it, use it for practice and experience. Assisting other established make-up artists is another way to gain experience.

Character make-up for film and television

This is totally different to the make-up used in the theatre, because cameras are involved. The newest, high intensity cameras are very critical of make-up and pick up every detail.

Most character make-up created for film and television is done using latex or prosthetics. For some of the major films, the research and the making of the prosthetic pieces may take up to one year to prepare. This book will not go into detail about prosthetics or characters using latex. That field of make-up is far too technical and involved. However, I will give you a brief outline of the two different styles.

Latex

Latex, which is actually liquid rubber, can be bought in any of the professional shops. Stippling is the method used when applying latex. You have to be very careful when handling these types of products, so I would suggest the best place to practise is on the hand. When you are proficient, then experiment on the face. Most areas on the face require two make-up artists to apply the product – one to stretch the skin while the other applies the product. Let's take the hand as a basic example of how to age with latex.

STEP by STEP

1. The person having the product applied can assist in the application by bending every joint in the hand, especially the wrist, to its maximum. This stretches the skin which, in turn, makes the ageing process more effective.
2. The fingers must be kept apart. If the latex touches while it is still tacky, it will stick together.
3. If the latex is being applied to a man, the hair is sometimes removed beforehand – otherwise, when the product is removed, it may pull out any hair in that area.
4. With the hand in this position, the latex is stippled over the entire area except the finger nails.
5. A single layer of tissue placed over the latex will add another 50 years to the overall effect. Some artists use cottonwool to achieve this effect, but this can be quite difficult at first. Break the tissue carefully between each finger and remove the excess edges. The tissue will dry the latex so that the second layer can be applied without the first being dried off with a hair dryer.
6. A second layer of latex is stippled over the tissue. This layer must be dried off completely with the hair dryer.
7. Once the latex is dry, details of ageing, such as liver spots and colouring, can be applied. The best product to use over latex is called rubber mask grease. This looks like a slightly softer version of a wax foundation and is stippled onto the latex. The detail should be drawn with a sable brush.
8. The hand is set by stippling powder on with a puff.
9. Finally, the hand is straightened, revealing the effect that latex gives when used in ageing.

Prosthetics

This is used when much more detail is required, or a particular shape needs to be created. A good example of prosthetics would be the character portrayed by the actor John Hurt in the film *The Elephant Man*. Christopher Tucker designed and applied the make-up for this character. Because of the distorted bone structure, the cast was sculpted on the actor's face to ensure it was comfortable enough to wear. The underlying sections were modelled in silicone rubber on a separate cast and the outer sections were done separately. It took many sections to make the head, all of which, when put together, had to appear totally natural. Many variations of latex were used to create the right appearance for each section, making the overall effect very realistic.

There are many different methods used for creating special effects with make-up, most of which are designed by the make-up artists themselves. They also design their own make-up to work with. The Research Council of Make-up Artists (RCMA) is one of the more popular ranges which has been developed for film and television make-up.

Straight film and television

STEPS TO NOTE

- If applying make-up to a woman, all fourteen steps are followed.
- If working on a man, only the first five steps are necessary in most cases (when foundation is required), otherwise just powder is used to stop any shine coming through.

Straight is the term used to describe everyday make-up in the film and television industry – the type of make-up seen on a person reading the news or hosting a chat show. If used in a film, it will relate to present day styles (as in *Pretty Woman* with Julia Roberts and Richard Gere, for example). Straight make-up should reflect what the person would wear off screen in his or her everyday life. The make-up might also be applied according to the style of clothes the professional will be appearing in, but this would usually be something of a classic style. The techniques for this kind of make-up would be the straightforward methods used in the other make-up styles.

REMEMBER

It is important to check carefully that the base is completely dry – any shiny area would show up on the screen as though the person was perspiring.

Make-up for the male artist

This will depend entirely on what each individual requires. Take two examples from the shows that I worked on for Sky TV. The host for the morning programme only required some loose powder. His complexion was evenly tanned and therefore did not require the application of any foundation. Powder was essential, however, to make sure that the skin did not appear shiny and therefore look sweaty. The make-up for the evening news presenter was not so simple. I applied a thin layer of liquid foundation which required moisturizer underneath it to even out his skin tone. Because of his receding hairline, the foundation was extended slightly further back onto the top of his head. This was necessary as the powder was taken right over the top of his head and would not have built up properly without the foundation under it. Working on any man with a bald head is done in the same manner, with foundation and powder – otherwise the top of the head lights up and appears to have light reflecting from it at all angles.

REMEMBER

Any area of the body which is visible should have a little foundation and powder applied. Check the hands in particular or, on a woman, the neckline. It may not be obvious to the eye, but it certainly will be in a photograph or on screen.

Questions

1 What is the difference between day and evening make-up?

2 Can you categorize make-up into different styles?

3 As a woman gets older, should the foundation be applied more thickly or more thinly?

4 Does the make-up for black-and-white photography differ from that used in colour photography?

7
Ethnic make-up

KEY AREAS

At the end of this chapter you will know how to:

- Apply make-up to different colour skins

The range of skin types covered includes:

Black
Asian
Oriental

In this chapter, I will be looking at the different needs, if any, that the Oriental, Asian and Black face requires.

REMEMBER

Take each skin type one step at a time, exactly as we have done with every other style of make-up.

The majority of the make-up application is carried out using exactly the same techniques as for white skin. There is only one point in each that needs a little more attention.

POINTS TO NOTE

- With black skin, the most important aspect is colour – which ones to use so that they will show up. Also remember that there are far more variations in the tones of black skin than there are in white skin. It should not be surprising that many black skins will need a lighter foundation than that which would be chosen for a white skin
- With an Asian face, the skin tone will need the most attention as it is generally uneven due to hereditary factors and diet. The pigmentation is much darker around the hairline and the eyes.
- With the Oriental face, the eyes are the most important feature. However, in dealing with the eyes, the shape of the face will also be affected. Shading down the side of the nose from the eyebrow gives the illusion that the nose is more prominent which, in turn, will make the face appear narrower.

Black skin

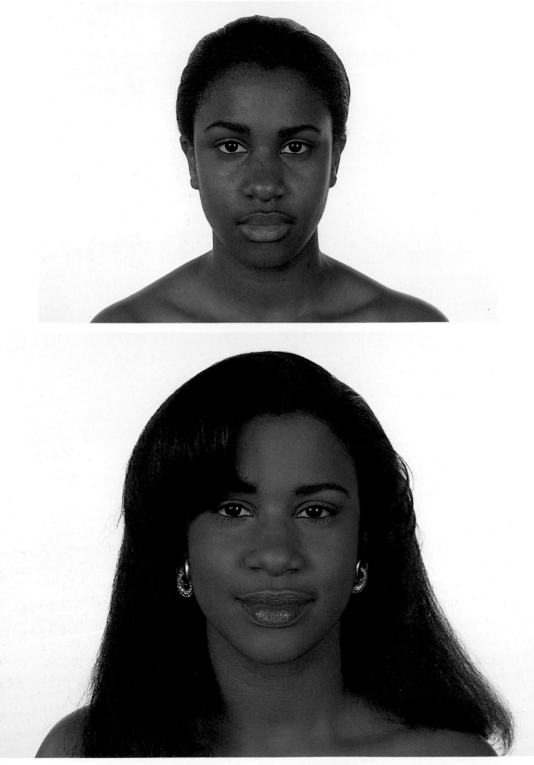

Day make-up

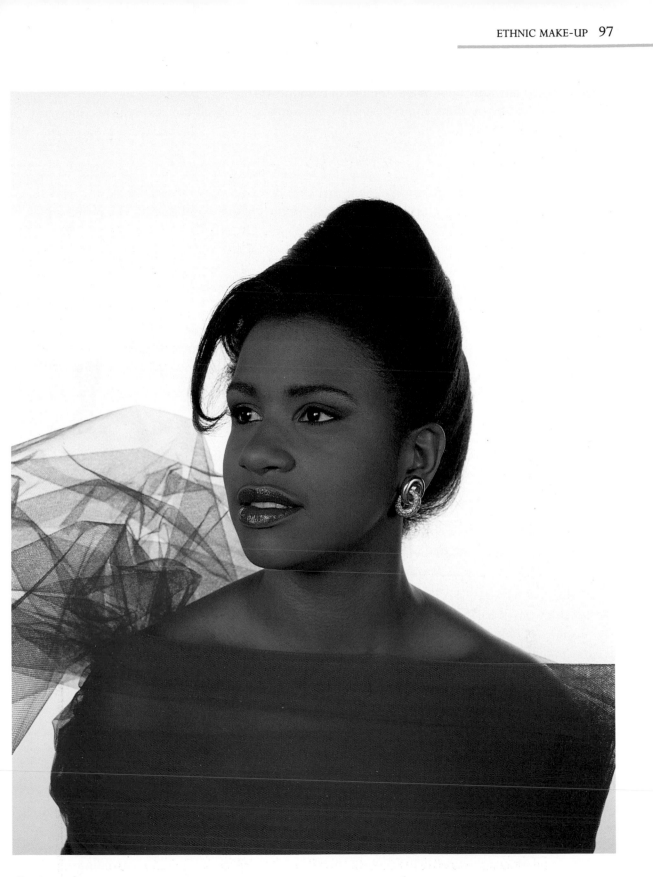

Evening make-up

Because we do not fully understand the use of colour, making up a black skin has often been shied away from. If you think about it sensibly, the application of all the cosmetic products is exactly the same on any face.

Products

The most obvious products to use are those that have been developed for black skin. Cosmetics for black skin are becoming more readily available in the chemists and stores. The professional ranges have always catered for all shades of skin.

Ordinary cosmetics can often be used, but you must check the amount of pigment they contain.

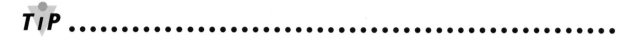

T*i*P •

Colour products like eyeshadow and blusher can be easily checked. Take a small amount of colour onto your finger — if it is the same colour which is in the compact, then that colour should be strong enough to show up on a black skin.

• •

Skin

The structure of black skin is completely different to that of white skin. The horny layer of a black skin is much thicker than that of a white skin. The sweat glands are also much larger and more numerous and, therefore, could affect the application of make-up and its staying power.

As white skin reflects the light, black skin absorbs it, which is why most of the black cosmetics available have a slight sheen to them. This glow to the skin should always be maintained, otherwise the skin may appear grey.

Foundation

Most black women have a perfectly even skin tone and therefore do not require foundation to even it out. A colourless base, like a tinted gel or moisturizer, is ideal for someone with a flawless complexion. If, however, the skin does need the coverage of a foundation, then a colour test is required to match the foundation to the skin tone. Remember that black skin includes many tone variations.

REMEMBER

One important point to note in testing for colour is that most black women prefer a shade of foundation slightly lighter than their skin tone.

The testing is done in exactly the same manner as for a white skin, just take the foundation which is a shade lighter. Many light-skinned black people can easily wear foundations which are designed for a white skin. I have often used a medium shade on a black skin, when I myself use dark. If foundations for white skin are used they should always be beige tones, avoiding any coloured pigment such as pink.

Powders

Because tinted powders for white skin contain substances like Titanium Oxide and Zinc Oxide, they cannot be used on a black skin without leaving a chalky, whitish residue. The powders for black skin are the best, or the alternative would be a totally colourless professional powder.

Colour

When dealing with colour products on a black skin, the choice of colour is easy as they all work well. It is the depth of colour which needs to be decided on carefully. Synthetic, natural or neutral; any of these colour combinations can be used. Until you are confident in working on black skin, I have listed some colour combinations below which can be used. Practise with these combinations and very soon you will have the confidence to make your own colour choice.

Colour combinations suitable for black skin

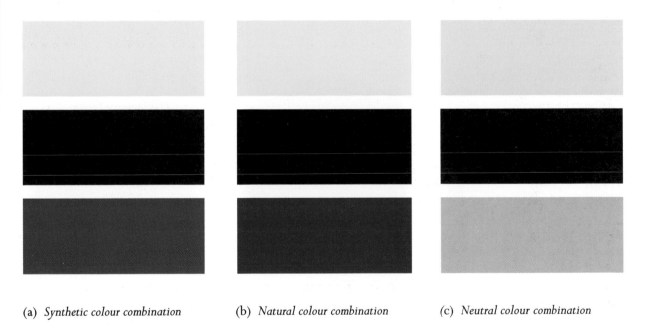

(a) *Synthetic colour combination*   (b) *Natural colour combination*   (c) *Neutral colour combination*

Lips

All black women have a double lip line which forms a raised area around the mouth. As most black lips are large, the inner line is always taken as the edge of the lips. Taking the lip colour to the outer edge would double the size of the mouth.

Eyes

Eyeliners and mascara are applied in the usual way. If false lashes are applied, strips would be the best style as black lashes are very curly. Singles would be too light and therefore pushed into the wrong position. This would not happen with strip lashes which are more solid.

Eyebrows

One other area which will need attention is the eyebrows. Because the hair is very curly, it may distort the shape of the eyebrow. The longer hairs at the end of the eyebrow may need removing completely so that a good shape can be drawn in. In most cases, black pencil alone is too dark. Draw the eyebrow in with brown first and then use the black to draw in tiny strokes which look like hairs.

Finishing touches

When the make-up is finished, do not forget to dust a little frosted powder over the skin. This will replace the natural glow which would have been removed when the translucent powder was applied.

Asian make-up

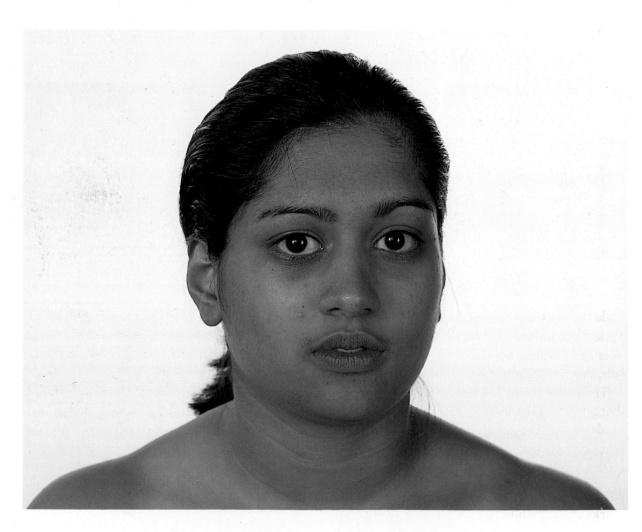

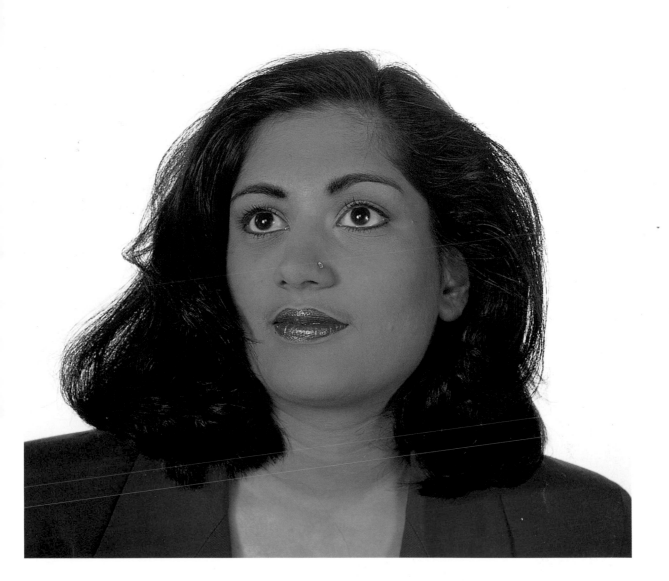

Make-up plays an important role in traditional Middle Eastern dress and can seem heavy by Western standards, especially the authentic wedding looks. The model above is wearing Western clothes, but you may well be working on a woman in traditional dress. In any country, hair, fashion and make-up should always be considered in creating the overall look.

There are no special features to be considered when making up an Asian face. The only area that needs particular attention is the skin. Due mainly to diet and hereditary factors, there is a tendency for the areas around the eyes and the mouth to be heavily pigmented.

Products

There are no special cosmetics to consider when dealing with an Asian skin. Treat it as though working on a white skin which is tanned.

Skin

The skin has yellow undertones. It is commonly believed that a pink foundation should be applied to counteract this, but this would in fact create an unnatural, mask-like appearance. Yellow skin tones can be neutralized by using synthetic colours on the eyes, cheeks and lips. Natural colours will, however, give a much more natural look, as shown in the example given.

Foundation

When choosing the foundation colour, the same rule applies as for black skin – pick a shade which is slightly lighter rather than darker. As a general rule it is appropriate to use paler foundation for a dark complexion and darker foundation for a white skin.

Because of the extra coverage needed to even out the skin tone, the best method to use for the foundation application would be the painting method. Apply one thin layer of foundation over the entire face and then apply a second layer in the areas which need extra coverage. If necessary, use two shades of foundation to achieve an even coverage. Work the foundation in well with the brush in the areas which need the extra coverage. The first layer of foundation which is applied should be very thin, otherwise it will become caked in the facial hair.

Eyebrows

Most Asian women have a lot of facial hair. Sometimes their hairline and eyebrows appear to be joined. A little of this may be removed above the eyebrows, but be careful not to remove too much.

Powder

Use a translucent powder containing no pigment as tinted powders will again leave a chalky, whitish residue.

Eyeliner

Traditionally, Asians wear eyeliner on the bottom lid as well as on the top lid. Always discuss this with your client before the mascara has been applied, and be prepared to be flexible in your approach.

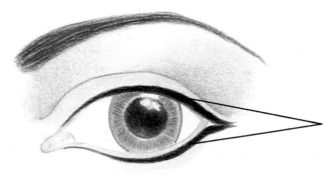

eyeliner, top and bottom

STEP *by* STEP

1. To apply eyeliner to the bottom lid, the head should be positioned straight with the eyes looking up to the ceiling.
2. Load a small eyeliner brush with liner and position the brush under the lashes. The full length of the hair should be in contact with the skin.
3. Pull the brush across the skin and a fine line will be revealed.
4. Reposition the brush at the inner corner of the eye and repeat the process until the two lines are joined.
5. At the outer corner of the eye, the top and bottom lines should be joined together.

Colour

When traditional dress is worn, the colours are quite vivid. So that the make-up can be seen against this background of bright colours, it may be necessary to finish off the eye make-up by adding a little vibrant colour over the top of the crease line. This is the position where we would normally apply a medium shadow. If the colours are too pale, the overall face will look washed out. This is where you will have to take your own initiative in deciding what looks right.

Oriental make-up

Skin tone and foundation

Oriental skin has many tone variations. The foundation colour is matched in the usual way – testing three colours across the forehead or any other clear section on the face. The most popular foundation in the humid climate of the Far East is Pan Cake. If this is what the client is used to, then using a colour test is not necessary as this product does not show any colour change. The colour which can be seen in the compact is how it will appear on the skin. Powder will also not be needed as this is already present in the foundation. Pan Cake is a very easy product to apply, usually with a damp sponge (see chapter 4). It can also be built up in areas which need extra coverage.

As the face can appear rather flat, a little shading is advisable underneath the cheek bones. Although in most cases (except theatrical make-up) I am against shading on the face because of its unnatural effect, it can be done in this instance using a slightly darker shade of foundation. This would work better if the foundation used was either a liquid or a cream texture. Work a little of the darker foundation on the underside of the cheek bone and blend it down so that it is not too obvious. This method can also be used on either side of the nose, to slim its wide appearance. Adding this slightly darker foundation will have to be done before any powder is applied. Applying shader this way creates a much more subtle effect than when it is applied over the powder.

Eyes

When working on an Oriental face, the attention should be focused on the eyes. Because of the bone structure of the Oriental face, it appears to show no socket line. This is a feature to take advantage of and emphasize. You can adapt the techniques already shown in this book to create a softer effect with a socket line. Refer to the diagram below for the position of each shadow colour and depth.

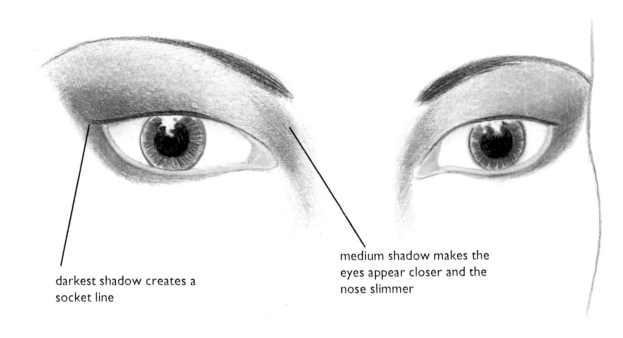

darkest shadow creates a socket line

medium shadow makes the eyes appear closer and the nose slimmer

Position of eyeshadow on an Oriental eye

Any of the techniques mentioned for applying shadow can be used. Particular attention should be taken with the eyelashes and the eyebrows, because Oriental hair has no bend in it. The eyebrows appear to grow outwards from the skin, which is why Oriental women usually cut them. The eyelash hair grows in a downward direction, which sometimes makes mascara difficult to apply. Strip false eyelashes are a better alternative.

Colour

The most flattering colours to choose for an Oriental skin are synthetic. In some cases neutral may be used, but in most instances stay clear of natural. For example, with the contrast of the white dress and the dark hair shown opposite in the photograph of an Oriental bride, synthetic shades are perfect. They will light up the face and counteract any yellow in the skin.

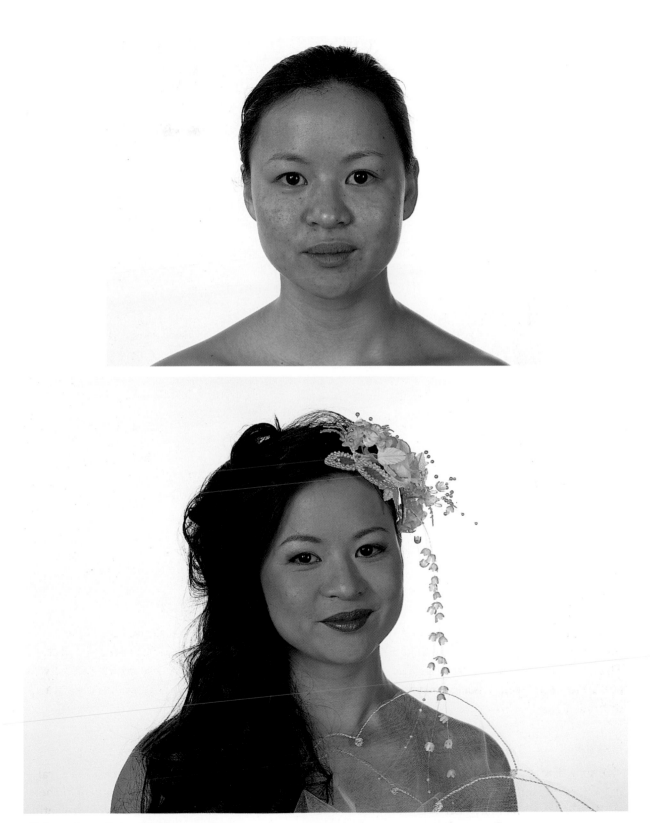

Make-up for an Oriental bride

By working to the guidelines shown throughout the book, you will have greater confidence to deal with any situation you are faced with — whatever colour, race or style. I wish you every success.

Questions

1 Can white cosmetics be used on a black skin?

2 Should a black skin be powdered until it is completely dry?

3 When applying make-up to an Asian client, which area should be paid particular attention to?

4 Which foundation texture is the best one to use in a hot, sticky climate?

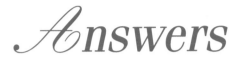

$\mathscr{A}$nswers

Chapter 1: Preparation

1 A compatible moisturizer is one which is totally absorbed into the skin, leaving no residue on the surface.

2 Oily skin should be prepared before the make-up with an anti-shine product or sealer.

3 Use an exfoliating cream to remove dry skin before applying any make-up products.

4 If the client is positioned at an angle when applying make-up, the shape of the bone structure will be distorted and the skin will be pulled in the wrong direction.

5 Always use a puff to stipple the powder onto a male model, as cotton wool will remain attached to the facial hair.

Chapter 2: Cosmetic products

1 Foundation is used to even out the skin tone and to create the base on which the colour products sit. It also protects the skin from the atmosphere.

2 Powder is used to absorb the oil content of the foundation and to create a dry surface for blending the colour products.

3 Blusher is used to give shape and colour to the face.

4 Lipstick can bleed due to body heat and use of a lipstick which is too soft.

5 Find the right foundation colour by doing the colour test. Apply different shades across the forehead (or any other clear area on the face). Allow the foundation a couple of minutes to dry to see if any colour change occurs.

Chapter 3: Tools of the trade

1 Retain the intensity of an eyeshadow by using a sponge-tipped applicator instead of a brush. Fifty per cent of the colour can be lost if it is applied with a brush.

2 There are three different hair shapes on professional brushes – flat top, hovis, and filbert. They vary in size by percentages or inches.

3 If wax or oily products have been used, the brushes can either be cleaned in a soapy solution or a solvent to dissolve the grease. Brushes should not be totally immersed in hot soapy water, just the actual hair.

Chapter 4: Application methods

1 Use an eyebrow pencil instead of a shadow to create a sharper, more fashionable finish to the eyebrow, and when working directly on the skin.

2 If mascara smudges, act immediately before the product dries. Take a cotton bud and point the tip directly onto the mascara. Rotate the bud between the thumb and the first finger, and the mascara will lift off immediately. If the product has dried, dampen the cotton bud.

3 Eyeshadow can be made to appear more vibrant by applying the same colour eye pencil underneath it.

4 Cover dark circles under the eyes by applying a second layer of foundation to the area. If the circles are very dark, use a slightly lighter shade of foundation or a highlighter.

5 Cover a scar or birthmark by applying a second layer of foundation with the painting brush.

6 Prevent eyeshadow from creasing by ensuring that the foundation creases are blended out well before applying powder.

Chapter 5: Colour and light

1 Make the eyes appear larger by using a darker eyeshadow. Be careful not to over-blend dark shadow, particularly on the bottom lid. Keep it sharp and clean.

2 Colour can be divided into two categories – natural and synthetic, or warm and cold.

3 The colours should always co-ordinate on the lips and cheeks.

4 Never use vibrant colours on an older face, stick to neutral colours.

Chapter 6: Make-up styles

1 There is very little difference between day and evening make-up. Most women have a style of make-up which they prefer. To apply something much heavier for the evening can sometimes make them uncomfortable. Eyeliner or false lashes will turn a day make-up into a more glamorous evening make-up.

2 It is impossible to categorize styles of make-up as each individual person or look requires something completely different, depending on age, colour or style.

3 As a woman matures the foundation should be applied as thinly as possible. A thicker foundation will emphasize age lines.

4 The main point to consider when applying make-up for a black-and-white photograph is contrast. White, black and grey shades are all that will be seen. As long as there is contrast between the skin and the colour areas, the make-up will work equally well for colour and black-and-white photography.

Chapter 7: Ethnic make-up

1 Colour cosmetics from a white range can be used on a black skin if the pigment in them is strong enough. It is, however, best to use a foundation from a range specifically for black skin, or one of the professional ranges like RCMA which has a vast range of foundations for every skin colour.

2 If a black skin is over-powdered, it will appear to have a grey tinge. When the make-up is completely finished, a light dusting of frosted powder will bring back the natural glow without leaving the skin tacky.

3 The main area to pay attention to when working on an Asian client is the foundation, due to uneven skin pigmentation and excessive facial hair.

4 The best foundation to wear in a hot, sticky climate is Pan Cake (foundation and powder mixed together). Any foundation which is tacky will feel uncomfortable on the skin and may disappear very quickly.

About the author

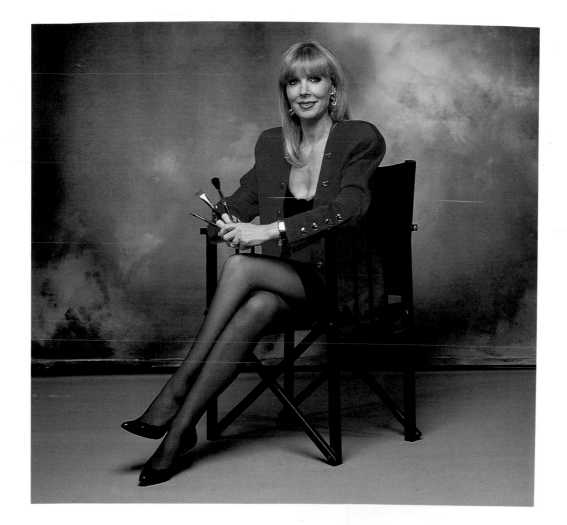

Linda Meredith has extensive experience in teaching make-up and her school, the International School of Make-up, offers short courses throughout the world to students who wish to perfect their make-up skills. The simplicity of her teaching methods has earned her recognition from many of the leading beauty associations and she is in great demand as a lecturer on the art of professional make-up. Linda firmly believes that any aspect of make-up taught should draw on practical experience. To back up her teaching techniques, Linda is still active in the field of professional make-up, often working on photographic shoots as well as teaching make-up to some of her famous clients. When Sky TV was launched, Linda ran their west-end make-up studios for the first year to perfect her skills in television make-up. Many of Linda's past students are working successfully as professional make-up artists. Self-motivation and determination are the keys to their success, with a little help from Linda.

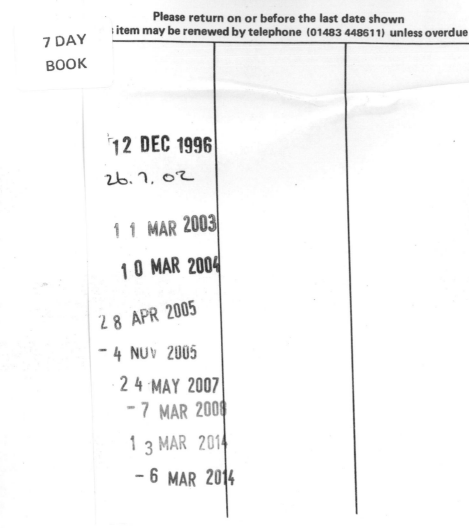